Copyright © 2026 by Foroogh Abinema.

All rights reserved. No part of this publication may be reproduced, distributed, or transmitted in any form or by any means, including photocopying, recording, or other electronic or mechanical methods, without the prior written permission of the publisher, except in the case of brief quotations embodied in critical reviews and other noncommercial uses permitted by copyright law.

ISBN: 979-8-9934667-1-2

Published by: Foro Wellness
https://sites.google.com/view/foro-wellness/home.

Cover design and back cover design by Erik Barona

Disclaimer

This book is intended for informational and educational purposes only. It is not intended as, and should not be considered, a substitute for professional medical, psychological, therapeutic, or health advice, diagnosis, or treatment. Always seek the advice of a qualified professional regarding any questions you may have about your health or well-being.

Printed in the United States of America.

TABLE OF CONTENTS

Acknowledgements 9
Foreword 1
Chapter 1 1
Introduction and Embracing Change 1
   Comparing Life Journey to Seasonal Experiences 2
   The First Spring Season of Life: 2
   The Summer Season of Life 6
   The Autumn Season of Life 9
   The Winter Season of Life 12
   The Second Spring Season of Life 14
Chapter 2 18
Young Adults Lifestyle Review 18
Chapter 3 23
Self-Awareness And Changing Lifestyle Habits 23
   Simple Stress Reliever Techniques 26
   Changing Our Food and Lifestyle Perception 30
   Overcoming Negative Belief 32
   Let Us Delve Into Self-Reflection 32
   Meditate and Quiet the Mind 34
   Table 1. 36
   Questioning Thoughts on The Mind 36
   Table 2: 37
   Practice Example to Take Action for Mind Shift 37

Chapter 4 41
Build a Participatory Resilience Perception Action
Challenge 41
    Independence and Autonomy 41
    Personal Growth and Learning 42
    Career Opportunities and Building Social Connections 42
    Balanced Diet and Nutritional Habits and Lifestyle
    Factors 43
    Relaxation And Meditation 45
    Social Connections 46
    Limit Alcohol and Avoid Substance Abuse 47
    Regular Health Check-ups 48
    Time Management 48
    Continuous Learning 48
    Setting Goals for Lifestyle Habits 49
    The Map of Participatory Wellness Action Plan 51
    Diagram1 52
    The Participatory Cycle of Wellness Change 52
    Practical Strategies For Building Resilience 54
Chapter 5 56
Recipes 59
    Olives And Oil Extracted from Olives 59
    Vegan Alternative To Eggs 60
    Chickpea Flour (Bean or Gram Flour) 61
    Legume Scramble 61

Nutritional Yeast	61
Herbal Cutlet Squares (Gluten-Free)	63
Spicy Herbal Scramble Egg	67
Spicy Tempeh Pumpkin Seed and Hazelnut Scramble (Vegan Option)	70
Spicy Scrambled Tempeh Wrap With Quinoa Bread	73
Egg Salad With Green Olives	76
Vegetable Omelet	80
Lemon Zest Quinoa Salad	84
Mom's Hearty Soup	87
Bean Soup	91
Carrot And Porridge Soup	95
Tortilla Coconut Tofu Cubes	98
Mushroom and Tofu Stew	102
Garlic Avocado Pesto	105
Mushroom Omelet	108
Lemony Shiitake Stew	112
Heavenly Saffron Steamed Basmati Rice	117
Nutty Split Pea Stew	121
Spicy Red Lentil Stew	126
Chili Veggie Style	130
Asparagus Soup	134
Mushroom Burger	138
Eggplant Tofu Stew	142
Herbal Nutty Pesto Spread	147

- Hazel Nut, Pumpkin Seed, and Herbal Tempeh Salad 151
- Homemade Berry Ice Cream 155
- Fruit Salad With Homemade Carrot Jam and Alternative Cream 158
- Carrot Jam 162
- Alternative to Cream 165
- Coconut, Oat, Banana Nut Cookies 168
- Mixed Nut Paste 171
- Nut Cookie Pastry 173
- Blueberry and Banana Scones 177
- Gluten-free Banana Cookies 180
- Gluten-Free Blueberry and Raisin Scones 183
- Homemade Organic Sourdough Bread 186
- Homemade Pizza with Tofu Cheese 189
- Homemade Nut Bar 193
- Chocolate Delight Bites 196
- Homemade Hummus 199
- Vegetarian Samosa 202

Summary 205

References 211

Acknowledgements

I want to express my gratitude to my mom and my beloved dad, may his soul rest in peace, whose unwavering love and support have been the foundation of my life's journey. To my loving husband, thank you for your hard work, encouragement, and wisdom, which have enriched our family. To my children, thank you for your love and for empowering me to share my message with the world.

I am writing to express special thanks to Dr. Keerthy for graciously taking the time to write the foreword for this book. Your continuous kindness, support, wisdom, and professional guidance have given me the courage to pursue my purpose, and I am truly honored to have you in my life journey.

I sincerely thank my son-in-law, Erik Barona, for his Incredible cover design. Your creativity and artistic talent are unique. Thank you for your dedication and support.

I thank my sisters, family, and friends worldwide. Each of you has impacted my life in ways I cannot fully express, and your support has meant the world to me. Thank you all for being a part of my story.

Foreword

Welcome to "Embrace the Young You" — a transformative guide that invites our youth to unlock their potential through the power of health, humanity, and mindful eating. Written by Foroogh Abinema, a passionate advocate for holistic well-being, this book is more than just a health challenge; it's an exciting adventure to discover the energy within you and learn how food, exercise, and compassion can fuel a healthier, happier life.

The journey begins with a deep dive into the essential lessons of life, where we reflect on personal experiences and explore how small choices can have a profound impact. You will learn the importance of becoming self-aware in today's technologically challenging world of today. You'll find inspiration in the stories of humanity in action — examples of how caring for others and connecting with the world around you lead to greater health and well-being. Through a blend of ancient wisdom from both Western and Eastern traditions, you'll discover powerful tools passed down through generations.

But this is not just about learning — it's about doing. With the Participatory Resilience Perception Action Challenge, you'll be empowered to create your own action plan, filled with plant-rich foods that nourish both body and soul. You'll see food not just as fuel, but also as a connection to the world around you and as a key to unlocking your inner power. The Vegan and Vegetarian Recipe section will guide you step by step, allowing you to take control of your health in a fun, meaningful, and purposeful way. I have been fortunate enough to try many of her recipes and have found them very easy and invigorating for my ongoing health journey. She is one of the world's most savvy and seasoned Chefs for healthy eating today.

As you embark on this journey, you'll not only discover a new way of eating but also a more profound sense of humanity, wisdom, and vitality. You are capable of amazing things, and through this challenge, you'll realize the power that lies within you. You will learn to design a map of action plans that you can use to solve lifestyle-related issues and find practical solutions to tackle a problem in your life.

So, take a deep breath, open this book with an open heart, and get ready to ignite your inner power. The next few weeks could change your life — one delicious, mindful, nutritious bite at a time.

With joy and excitement for your journey,

Namaste

Keerthy Sunder, M.D.

Amazon Best Selling Author-Face Your Addiction & Save Your Life

Chief Medical Officer, Karma Doctors & Associates, California

Chapter 1
Introduction and Embracing Change

Being young is a fantastic stage of life's journey, yet it also carries significant uncertainty. Having left home and moved to a new country at eighteen, I understand how tough and uncertain young adults feel as they step into a new phase of their lives. As a mother of two, I also experienced how my young adult children had to do the same: leave home to pursue a new chapter of their lives, moving away from their familiar environment to attend university or take a new job in a different city or country. I faced many of the same challenges they did, which gave me a deeper understanding of how delicate this stage of life can be without the proper support and guidance. That realization motivated me to enroll in a health research program to address the challenges young adults face, particularly those related to health and well-being. I aim to share my research findings and my own experience to develop practical solutions to the barriers I've identified in young adults' efforts to become independent.

I aim to encourage innovative approaches to overcoming obstacles and provide straightforward solutions that promote well-being. I am sharing my experience in nutrition and health in the hope that it will positively influence your lives and help you make the world a better place for yourselves and future generations. As dietitians, we provide our clients with practical solutions for diet and lifestyle changes. I am including simple vegetarian recipes and vegan options to support your food and lifestyle choices and help you along your journey. I include vegetarian recipes to support the health benefits of incorporating more plant-rich foods and to save money. I realize that some individuals are vegetarians and vegans because of ethical issues, and I respect that, too. The diet and lifestyle information is for general educational purposes only and does not replace your health practitioner's advice.

Comparing Life Journey to Seasonal Experiences

As we move through the stages of our lives, we can compare each stage to seasonal changes in nature. Since different seasons in nature bring about various changes and opportunities, similar changes occur throughout our lives. We look, feel, and desire different things at different stages of our life cycle.

The First Spring Season of Life:

Spring is a time when nature is full of new growth and rejuvenation, and similarly, childhood has that sense of excitement and curiosity about the world around us. Children are often eager to explore, learn, and discover, much like how nature comes alive in spring. Similarly, childhood is a period of continuous development and unfolding. Children undergo various stages of physical, emotional, and intellectual growth, much like the changing seasons. I am comparing childhood to the first spring, a time filled with the promise of new beginnings, exploration, and the joy of discovery.

It captures the essence of the curiosity, excitement, and continuous growth that characterize the early years of life, much like the refreshing, rejuvenating qualities of spring. Just as spring brings a sense of renewal and freshness to nature with the blossoming of flowers and the emergence of new leaves, a similar sense of novelty often characterizes childhood. Everything is new to a child and the world around them. There is a sense of excitement and curiosity.

Of course, childhood development is different for each child. Your upbringing can be influenced by where you live and your family circumstances. As a child, your family, friends, schoolmates, teachers, the outside environment, and the media all influence you.

Looking back, it is incredible how one of my childhood experiences redirected my life and deepened my connection to natural and holistic food and medicine. My mother shared a memory from when I was just a few months old. It was a moment no one expected. A family member tried to lift me and, in doing so, dislocated my left shoulder. After that incident, my mother noticed something was wrong with my left arm. My mom was alarmed because I couldn't hold it up, and it would fall. She took me to so many pediatric doctors, and they all told her I was born that way and that they could do nothing for me. My mother, bless her heart, persisted and found a natural healer. He had a natural cream and instructed my mom to make a poultice and continue using it for a few weeks. After a while, my arm began to heal, and my mother, as she explained, began to calm down. I am very grateful to my mother for not giving up on me and to the healer who helped heal my arm. I now understand why I am drawn to natural herbs, food, and remedies.

Another time was when my family suffered from food poisoning due to consuming fish that had been in waters contaminated by an oil tank spillage, except my younger sister, who did not have the fish dish, from what I recall. The doctor made a house call, and when he examined all of us who were sick, he said that I had to be admitted to the nearby hospital. I remember being worried as I was the only one who had to go to a hospital out of my family. I was there for nearly a week. When I went back home and had a follow-up with my general practitioner, he teased me since he knew I was the only one out of our family who was admitted to the hospital. He asked, "What happened? Did you eat more than your family to end up in the hospital?" Thank goodness we all recovered from that incident. Being young, one recovers from illnesses and injuries so fast.

I can share some joyful childhood memories from summer holidays and New Year celebrations when I was eight or nine. I used to look forward to the new year, seeing relatives, visiting family and friends, exchanging gifts, and wearing new clothes and shoes. During the summer holidays, we would travel to Southwest Iran to visit relatives and experience our family's unconditional love. I would wake up to the natural alarm clock of neighborhood roosters and watch my grandma, bless her soul, bake fresh sourdough bread in her open-flame oven in her small courtyard. Her kitchen was simple, with no modern appliances—only a small stove and a table. They would prepare everything from scratch.

Some afternoons during the holiday, they would bake cookies, and the smell of freshly baked cookies would fill the air. Then, guests would come for afternoon tea. They had a substantial, tall date tree in their yard. God bless my grandpa's soul and his agile stamina. He would climb the tree to cut some dates and bring them down quickly. These scenes are vividly etched in my memory. One of my dad's relatives had a citrus fruit grove. Oh, how magical it was to go there to play, pick fruit, and share it with family and friends.

I am grateful for these happy memories and for navigating tough times with positive outcomes. I realize there are many ups and downs, and not everyone has many happy childhood memories. Looking back, whether you had a happy childhood or a not-so-happy one, you would still know that the next season was coming, and there is a sense of innocence and hope associated with the first spring of your life.

We all face numerous challenges, and our parents or caretakers will undoubtedly do their best to protect and provide a safe environment for our childhood. I have heard clients mention that they had a tough childhood, and sometimes their parents and caregivers did not provide the optimal care and environment for their children. I have come to realize that everyone's actions and way of thinking are shaped by what they know at the time. By reassessing this fact, we can come to terms with individuals and incidents that have caused hurt feelings in the past. Recognizing that we are all constantly changing and learning from our experiences, we can let go of resentment toward someone or a situation, which can bring relief. Letting go, in a way, frees us from attachment to feelings that do not benefit us and, at times, are a burden.

The Summer Season of Life:

Adolescence, through the mid-twenties, can be considered the summer season of one's life. Summer is a season of warmth, but also occasional ups and downs. Similarly, the period from adolescence to the mid-twenties is recognized as a time of uncertainty and opportunity. You face numerous challenges and must make decisions about education, career paths, and personal relationships. It is a vibrant and transformative time, filled with possibilities, self-exploration, and the potential to make meaningful contributions to the world. It captures the essence of this phase as a season of personal and professional growth, much like the energy and dynamism of summer. This season of life is the time to explore and discover your talents. You are curious about travel, thinking, and imagining the opportunities and careers that await you. It is like being in high school and daydreaming about what you want to do during the summer holidays—wondering in the back of your mind about opportunities and, at the same time, uncertainties. It's a time to ponder personal goals, values, and aspirations, much like the reflective moments one might have during summer. It is a time of uncertainties and opportunities. It's a reasonable time to consider how to utilize your talents and ambitions. It emphasizes the potential for making a positive impact on a broader scale.

My mid-twenties were a challenging time. I moved to the United Kingdom to further my education and had to prepare to study English and attend university. At times, I felt inadequate because of the language barrier and being away from home in a foreign country. I had to go to the embassy every year to renew my visa. My sisters and I even had to register with the local police station wherever we lived. One Sunday, I recall looking out my dorm room window and seeing two tall policemen walking on the grounds. I wondered what it was all about. Shortly after, I heard a knock on my door. I opened it, and to my surprise, the two policemen were standing by my door!

I was worried and scared, to be honest. The police officers explained that my sister and I had not informed them of our latest address change, and that this was a friendly reminder. It was embarrassing to go through all that because we had done nothing wrong, only because of the countries' political situations. It is tough to encounter these incidents when we have done nothing wrong. I lived in a dorm for two years, and most people in similar age groups had a lot of free time. They certainly had fun and attended parties every weekend. My sister and I were living in the same dorm. We were majoring in science, which meant we didn't have as much free time as we'd like because we had to study. The embarrassing moments I remember were when a few residents in the dorm would ask us at the breakfast table some mornings if we had gone out the night before or which party we planned to attend over the weekend. The first few times, we answered that we had no plans to attend parties because we had to study; they looked at us as if we were from another planet. Then, after a while, we realized we just had to present them with more exciting stories and adventures so they wouldn't look at us strangely. It was a tough time, as for eight years back home, our country was at war. Our parents had to move from our hometown because it was in a war zone from 1980 to 1988. They had to start their lives over in a new city. The entire family was affected by that. We had to work harder to appreciate how hard our parents worked to support us, even during tough times of war. Although that period of my life was challenging and marked by many ups and downs, the youthful energy kept me going, and there was always room to be grateful for the survival of innocent people and the new opportunities that arose in my life.

The Autumn Season of Life:

Natural changes, such as crop harvesting and leaf shedding, characterize the autumn season. The analogy suggests that this phase of life is when one reaps the rewards of earlier efforts, makes choices, and experiences change.

In the same way, autumn is a harvest season; this life phase is a time to gather the fruits of one's efforts. It may involve reaping the benefits of educational and career pursuits, as well as personal growth and the development of skills and experiences.

You pursue a career and a job, emphasizing the importance of establishing independence during this phase. It's a time when individuals focus on building a stable foundation for their professional lives and personal autonomy. This phase may involve building personal relationships, starting a family, and taking on additional responsibilities. During this time, individuals often struggle to balance their personal and professional lives.

Autumn is a season of change, and this life phase may involve reflection and adjustments. Individuals may reassess their goals, values, and priorities and make necessary changes to align with their circumstances. Autumn is often associated with maturation, and the mid-twenties to mid-thirties are a period of increased responsibility and maturity. During this time, individuals may assume leadership roles, make significant life decisions, and contribute to others' well-being. Autumn marks the transition from summer's vibrancy to winter's quiet preparation. Similarly, this life phase signifies a shift from the energetic pursuits of youth to a more settled, purposeful approach, preparing for the next stages of life.

It captures the idea of reaping the rewards of earlier efforts, establishing independence, and navigating the responsibilities of career, family, and personal growth. This phase is a time of transition, reflection, and preparation for the chapters of life that follow.

My journey during this season of my life had its challenges. I married in my late twenties and had to wait two years for my permit to join my husband, who was living in America. I lived in the UK, and my husband was in the USA. My husband had only two weeks of vacation per year, so we could see each other for only two weeks out of the year for the first two years of our marriage! Life has many ups and downs, and with my optimistic nature, I continued to seek out positive experiences and remained grateful. Then, I had two children in my early thirties. I had some family support when we lived in the United Kingdom. Then we moved to different countries due to my husband's job relocation. Establishing my family in new countries and moving every four years or so was challenging. Reflecting on those difficult times has made me more resilient in dealing with life's challenges. I guess the German philosopher Friedrich Nietzsche was right over a century ago when he said, "Out of life's school of war, what doesn't kill me makes me stronger." I would perhaps not emphasize war and use a simpler version of that expression to 'Out of life's school, what doesn't kill me makes me stronger."

I lived in Alaska for ten years. I have beautiful memories of Alaska, but I also remember the challenging times. I was far from family and friends, and I remember the long flights to see them and the harsh winters. By around October, one must be prepared for the seven months ahead, whatever the weather has in store for us. By around May, everyone emerges from hibernation and looks forward to the long summer days. While I lived in Alaska, we experienced several earthquakes, including one in the middle of the night. My husband was on a business trip, and I was at home with my two small children. I immediately brought them to my side, and we all cuddled until the shaking stopped. It was scary, but I tried to be brave for the children's sake and showed strength. My kind neighbor called me, comforting me with the thought that someone was looking out for us. I must admit that my experience in Alaska was one of a kind. Even though the terrain was harsh and cold, the people were kind-hearted and friendly, bringing warmth to our lives.

The Winter Season of Life:

The mid-thirties to mid-forties can be seen as the winter season of our lives. Winter is often associated with quiet reflection, cooler temperatures, and a sense of maturity. Similarly, the analogy suggests that this phase of life is a time of continued responsibilities and challenges, when individuals may approach life with a more seasoned, cautious perspective.

You may be immersed in career responsibilities, financial commitments, and the day-to-day challenges of managing a household and family. Winter is a season that often calls for caution and preparedness because of challenging weather conditions. Similarly, this life phase may call for a more cautious approach to decision-making, informed by accumulated experience and lessons learned over the years.

Creating an independent life suggests that you have already laid a foundation for yourself in this phase. It's a time when personal and professional achievements contribute to a sense of independence and self-reliance.

This phase often involves taking care of yourself and assuming responsibility for your family's well-being. You may navigate the challenges and joys of parenthood, focusing on your children's needs and development. The analogy highlights winter as a time of caregiving and nurturing, much like the season's need for warmth and protection. You may prioritize your children's and family members' well-being by offering support and guidance. Winter is a time for introspection, and this phase may involve reflection and inner growth. You may reassess your personal goals, values, and priorities to align them with changes in your life.

Winter is a season of preparation for the eventual renewal of spring. Similarly, this life phase may involve preparing for the next stages, whether planning for children's education, retirement, or other future endeavors. The winter season is often compared to the mid-thirties to mid-forties, a time of continued responsibility, cautious decision-making, and nurturing relationships. At this time, you often find fulfillment in caring for your family, maintaining your independence, reflecting on personal growth, and preparing for the future.

I was fortunate to have a promising career that allowed me to return to school when my children were in kindergarten and primary school. I pursued further education with the support of my family while living in the United Kingdom. It was tough balancing work, studying, and caring for my family, but I managed to do so. Although I had to leave my established permanent position because of my husband's frequent relocations, I found new jobs in each new country after settling the family into the new environment. As I reflect on my adult children's lives, I see that both earned their master's degrees while working full-time in their early thirties. I witnessed how hard they both worked, balancing full-time work, personal life, and their studies.

By reflecting on our life experiences and these seasons, we must take action and seize the opportunities life presents.

The Second Spring Season of Life:

In your mid-forties, you enter a phase marked by introspection and self-discovery. This season of life is when you often reflect on the various aspects of your life. Questions about what makes you happy and the critical values in life signal a deep introspection into personal fulfillment and priorities. You may reflect on what brings you joy and align your life with its most significant values. You begin to view life from a wider lens and a broader perspective. This is because, with age and experience, individuals gain a more comprehensive view of their lives and the world around them. When I compare this phase to a second spring, it is because there is a sense of renewal, growth, and vibrancy. Just as spring represents a time of natural rejuvenation, it is also an opportunity for personal renewal and exploration. Spring is often associated with new beginnings, and this phase is an opportunity for personal and professional reinvention. You may reassess your goals and aspirations and welcome new opportunities as they arise. The comparison to spring suggests a joyous embrace of change and growth. It's a time when you may be open to changes in your life, whether in relationships, career, or personal pursuits. Spring is a season of blooming flowers and vibrant colors.

Similarly, this phase may involve reconnecting with passions and interests that may have taken a back seat during earlier life stages. The metaphor suggests a balance between the wisdom gained through experience and the enthusiasm that comes with a renewed sense of purpose. It's a time when you may draw on your accumulated knowledge to make informed decisions. The mid-forties to mid-sixties are a time of reflection, self-discovery, and renewed enthusiasm—akin to experiencing a second Spring in life's journey. It's a phase marked by asking fundamental questions about happiness and values, embracing change, and viewing life through a broader lens.

From my life experience, I realized there is a reason they say life begins in your forties! To me, it felt like a new beginning, as my perspective on life had shifted. As I approached my forties, I felt liberated from life's resistance. It was as if time had come again to rediscover myself with less friction. It felt like entering another springtime of life. I rediscovered myself and saw the world from a different perspective. I felt that I did not need to prioritize anyone's approval over my own life decisions. I began to appreciate myself and value my intuition and inner strength.

I lost my dear father in my fifties, and the way I learned to cope with emotional loss was to tap into my inner soul strength. That transformation strengthened me and awakened my purpose to share life lessons and experiences and to serve the world by spreading my message. I began to see the world from a different perspective. Reflecting on life's hardships strengthens you. As one enters the fifties and sixties, approaches retirement, and beyond, there is an opportunity to relearn, spend time with grandchildren, and find joy in the new generations. You can embrace life's simple pleasures with children and grandchildren, and, if you're lucky, with great-grandchildren. This book aims to help you discover your inner wisdom sooner.

In summary, the sooner you begin reflecting on your life, on what brings you happiness, and on how you can serve the world through your passions, the faster you will discover the new spring season of your life.

Of course, each season of life can bring different experiences to different individuals. The quality of your experiences depends on your circumstances. My goal in this book is to foster positive energy and appreciation for you, helping you recognize your full potential and navigate life's challenges.

As I enter the second spring of my life, I want to remind younger generations, through this book, that you can choose to experience the warmth of spring, rejuvenation, and rebirth in any season of your life. There is great joy in tapping into one's creativity by learning from life experiences and in the transformative changes that can occur when one listens to and trusts one's body's wisdom, thereby making one's life a great story.

Chapter 2

Lifestyle Review of Early Adulthood

Many thoughts run through a young adult's mind: moving away from home, finding a place to live, managing finances, organizing time, and navigating new social situations. The responsibilities of living independently, handling money, and pursuing education or a career can increase anxiety and stress. Financial pressure can be overwhelming, especially when you realize you need to budget for daily expenses, food, rent, and unexpected costs. Additionally, adjusting to a new social environment, making friends, and building a social network can take time and effort. Learning effective time management is essential. For instance, balancing time for schoolwork, a job, and personal life can be intimidating.

Additionally, tasks include daily chores such as cleaning, cooking, laundry, and repairs, as well as saving money. These new responsibilities and inadequate sleep can affect cognitive function and emotional well-being.

This chapter reviews research on key lifestyle issues. I will examine the realities, but I want to reassure you now that the following chapters will provide solutions and empowering messages. I'm sharing these findings so you have the facts. Whether you are at that age or know a family member or friend going through that life phase, this information can be helpful.

The period from adolescence to the mid-twenties is a turbulent, defining chapter, marked by the transition from home to a new phase of life. It is an overwhelming transition to independence.

A young adult's mind is burdened with:

• Logistics of Independence: Finding a place to live and handling daily chores (cooking, cleaning, laundry, repairs).

• Financial Pressure: Budgeting for rent, food, and unexpected expenses can be overwhelming.

• Social Adaptation: Investing effort and time to form new friendships and establish a social circle.

• Time Management: Learning to balance school, work, personal life, and self-care is a daunting, essential skill.

This stress is often compounded by the pressure to achieve academic and career success. Furthermore, inadequate sleep is a common problem that significantly affects cognitive function and emotional well-being.

Diet, Weight, and Convenience:

In this era of convenience, comfort, and speed, young adults are particularly vulnerable to adopting unhealthy habits. Studies highlight a growing concern: obesity, driven by environmental factors that encourage the consumption of high-energy-dense foods and a decline in physical activity. The shift toward mass-prepared, highly processed food—loaded with sugars, fats, and flavor enhancers—is marketed brilliantly to a busy demographic. This culture has a clear effect:

• A U.K. survey of students found that 57% never cooked because of a lack of time, and 40% relied on convenience and ultra-processed foods, which are often high in added fat, sugar, and calories.

• When young adults gain independence (especially when entering university or starting a new job), they are exposed to a setting that can trigger weight gain.

In the U.S., about 30% of college students are overweight or obese. The much-discussed "Freshman 15" might be an exaggeration, but multiple studies agree that first-year students gain between four and nine pounds. This rapid weight gain is a significant health issue, as being overweight and obese are inflammatory conditions. It is a crucial time, as during these periods of life, you become more autonomous and establish lifelong habits. For many, this is their first attempt at independent living and managing their own dietary and lifestyle choices.

Unfortunately, poor lifestyle behaviors established between ages 18-35 often persist into later life, significantly increasing the risk of chronic disease.

The consequences are stark:

• Cardiovascular disease (CVD) risk factors are elevated in university students.

• A higher weight-to-height ratio during university is a predictor of subsequent diabetes.

• A study of young adults (aged 24–32) found that 69% were prehypertensive, and 27% were prediabetic.

These behaviors form the foundation for lifelong health. Since young adults often forgo routine medical checks, high blood pressure or blood glucose levels can go unnoticed.

I noticed these behaviors and issues when I was around young adults going through that phase of their lives. That is why I conducted research to identify solutions to share. My aim in reviewing these studies is to raise awareness of the problem and to present practical solutions.

Mental Health and Support:

Mental health among young adults is a pressing concern. Along with substance misuse, mental health disorders are the leading source of disability in this demographic in the United States. Nearly two-thirds of the disability burden in young adults stems from these two issues. By age 29, over half of all individuals have experienced such a disorder. The evidence points to a clear need: policies and programs that directly address the complex needs of young adults. Allocating resources for preventive mental health programs will help this generation succeed in education, employment, and social relationships, ultimately enhancing their overall well-being. But what if you or a friend is already struggling?

Knowing how to access professional support if you're dealing with substance misuse or a developing disorder is a vital, life-saving skill. It's crucial to know that strong support systems are available to you. Whether it's reaching out to a confidant, using a student health service, connecting with a medical professional, or finding community programs, you do not have to carry this burden alone. Help is always available, and asking for it is a sign of strength, not weakness.

Chapter 3

Self-Awareness and Changing Lifestyle Habits

This chapter offers a collection of simple, actionable strategies for navigating independent living. These solutions aren't just theory; they are grounded in my personal journey—stories of stumbling, learning, and cultivating self-awareness—and supported by relevant research and observations from the front lines of early independence. I will distill complex challenges into manageable, daily steps, giving you the practical tools you need to thrive on your own terms.

When we think of wellness, healthy habits often come to mind, encompassing optimal physical, emotional, mental, and social health. Through self-reflection and self-awareness, we can gain a deeper understanding of our emotional and cognitive well-being. Healthy habits are fundamental to a balanced lifestyle, which includes maintaining a healthy weight through nutrient-dense food choices, staying active, and nurturing our mental health. Various barriers and motivators influence our dietary habits.

For example, you might be considering living independently and pursuing further education or a career. Access to local supermarkets, the availability of physical training centers, and proximity to family are motivators for healthy weight-related behaviors. Barriers to healthy eating habits include a lack of practical nutritional knowledge and the availability of high-calorie, high-fat foods in your dorms and living environments. The literature indicates that being away from family, poor time management, and reduced physical activity are additional barriers to adopting a healthy lifestyle.

Furthermore, frequent consumption of fast food is also a barrier to maintaining a healthy weight. A systematic assessment of 187 countries concluded that, on average, older adults had better diets than younger adults. It also found that consumption of unhealthy foods had significantly increased. Improvements in healthier food choices were associated with higher national incomes, while wealthy countries also scored highly on unhealthy food consumption.

I remember living in a dorm in Scotland decades ago; we had a weekly set menu. I liked only some of the food we were served. Most options were either too salty, too sugary, or too oily, or contained meats I wouldn't eat, but that was what was available. My budget did not allow me to explore other options. I sometimes saved the bun from my morning breakfast and made a butter-and-jam sandwich for lunch, accompanied by a piece of fruit, since the dorm only provided breakfast and dinner. My intake could have been healthier if there had been more nutritious options or if my budget had allowed me to choose alternatives.

I could see the same situation with my adult children. Their diets were limited by the limited food options available in the dorm and at a nearby canteen. My daughter discovered ramen noodles while in college and admitted to relying on them during that time. My son asked me to write down some traditional Persian recipes in a notebook when he moved out of the dorm and rented an apartment with a few other friends. I was so glad to hear him ask for that. I wrote down some recipes for him, and he prepared meals based on them. He began preparing meals for the week.

I realized then that intervention at this stage could help reverse the trend of nutritional insufficiency and the consequent risk factors for chronic disease. By being aware of this information, you can help identify solutions to these risk factors. For example, if you live in a dorm, you can survey students' likes and dislikes. Then you can plan a menu around popular, healthier ingredients. In a way, you take responsibility for your health by participating in planning dorm menus alongside a university health professional.

Therefore, interventions in this age range would benefit society by considering young adults' culture and socioeconomic status and by exploring the factors that promote a more productive lifestyle. The solutions that come to mind include: effective time management, financial management, relaxation, maintaining a positive mindset, increasing physical activity, adopting healthier eating habits, fostering a sense of belonging, cultivating self-awareness, and establishing a supportive network. These strategies can help reduce the health risks associated with barriers to a healthy lifestyle.

Simple Stress Reliever Techniques

I would also like to rename "stress" to "overthinking." When searching for the meaning of stress and its origins, we come to understand that it is a human-made word that has acquired significance. It is a way of overthinking situations, and we make them ourselves.

Let us consider ways to empower ourselves to take greater control of environmental factors, reduce barriers, and capitalize on the positive aspects that foster good habits and a healthier lifestyle. When discussing time management, it is essential to include time for self-reflection and appreciation. Time spent on yourself and on being grateful for your body is also crucial to your health and happiness.

The innate powers of bodily systems to overcome stress: The vagus nerve is a vital component of the autonomic nervous system, which regulates numerous involuntary bodily functions. It plays a significant role in maintaining health through several mechanisms. For example, the vagus nerve helps regulate heart rate by transmitting signals that slow it, promoting a balanced, healthy cardiovascular system. It aids digestion by stimulating the production of digestive enzymes and promoting peristalsis, which moves food through the digestive tract.

The vagus nerve has anti-inflammatory effects. It helps regulate the immune response and can reduce inflammation, which is beneficial for preventing chronic diseases. It supports the parasympathetic nervous system, which is responsible for the "rest and digest" response, helping to reduce stress and anxiety. The vagus nerve can affect mood and emotional well-being by regulating the release of neurotransmitters, including serotonin. It can also influence breathing patterns, thereby improving respiratory health and facilitating efficient oxygen exchange.

Breathing technique:

We can be curious about the vital force of breathing and learn techniques to calm our nerves. Engage in slow, deep breathing exercises. Deep breaths stimulate the diaphragm, which, in turn, activates the vagus nerve, which helps relax the body's systems.

Your calmness is only a few breaths away. When you feel angry or frustrated, step away from the situation and focus on your breathing. For example, take nine deep breaths in and nine deep breaths out. Afterward, you will feel less angry or anxious. This simple breathwork technique can help you feel calmer and more centered.

Brief exposure to cold, such as splashing cold water on your face or taking a cold shower, can activate the vagus nerve, which triggers the parasympathetic nervous system and helps keep the body calm.

Vocalization and Sound and The Vagus Nerve:

I am sure you have encountered friends, family, or even yourself singing or humming in the shower, which brings a sense of happiness. There is a scientific reason for this. Singing stimulates the vagus nerve. So now you can tell your roommate there is a scientific reason for your humming and singing, and they won't tease you anymore.
The same effect occurs when vigorously gargling with water. Gargling activates our vocal cords, which, in turn, stimulates the vagus nerve.

Genuine laughter, especially belly laughter, stimulates the vagus nerve and can reduce stress. Other simple ways to stimulate the vagus nerve, promote relaxation, and reduce stress include physical activity, meditation, and massage.

Emerging evidence suggests a link between gut health and the vagus nerve. Consuming probiotics and maintaining a healthy gut microbiome may indirectly support vagal tone. I have included vegetarian and vegan recipe options in Chapter 5 that support the gut microbiome. What is the microbiome, I hear you ask. The term was introduced by Joshua Lederberg, who defined it as a community of microorganisms, including fungi, bacteria, viruses, and other microbes, in a particular environment. These microorganisms can live on our skin and in our gastrointestinal tract (gut). The health of these microorganisms affects our health. Vegetarian foods support a healthy gut microbiome, which is one of the reasons this guidebook includes vegetarian recipes.

Positive Social Interaction:

Being part of a community activates the vagus nerve. Hugging, bonding with loved ones, and connecting with them can activate the vagus nerve and reduce stress.

Interacting with nature, whether in your neighborhood or a nearby park, is a simple yet effective way to calm your nerves. As you walk, notice your breathing as you step forward with one foot, then the next, and then the next. Count your breaths in and out: take one step forward and breathe in, then take three steps and breathe out. Gradually increase the number of steps to a comfortable breathing rate.

When I think of calm, I picture walking barefoot along a beach and listening to the waves. Studies show that negative ions in the air near the sea or ocean can help balance our energy. Negative ions are oxygen atoms with an extra electron. They are naturally formed by water, air, sunlight, and the Earth's inherent radiation.

I learned about a stress-relief technique years ago. It is called the Emotional Freedom Technique (EFT) or tapping, a holistic practice that is easy to learn and apply to oneself. It produces relief from stress, anxiety, and the symptoms of burnout within minutes. Many websites, videos, and tutorials can teach you how to do it. The website I came across was created by Nick Ortner in 2007. The website (thetappingsolution.com) shows people how to relieve stress by pressing or tapping specific acupressure points and saying affirmations they wish to come true. The acupressure points for this practice are on the top of the head, by the eyebrows, by the eyes, under the eyes, under the nose, under the mouth, by the collarbone, under the arms, and on the sides of the hands. Use both hands to tap these pressure points while repeating the mantra you wish to change and make happen. For example, say, "Even though I feel this pain or anger or stress, name wherever your pain and feeling of anger are coming from." Keep tapping on all these pressure points, then say, "I can give my body permission to heal me and feel better, and become relieved of this pain, and indicate where the pain originates from." The literature notes that as you repeat this process, you will notice the pain, anger, or stress you felt before tapping has subsided to some degree. This is a simplified explanation; however, refer to the website I included for further information.

Changing Our Food and Lifestyle Perception:

According to Webster's Dictionary, a habit is a routine behavior that is repeated regularly and often occurs subconsciously. We are all creatures of habit, and by acknowledging this, we can find ways to improve them so they serve us better. After years of research, experiencing these challenges, and witnessing them in my children as they attended university away from home, I have designed this map to guide participation in empowered action plans. It aims to examine lifestyle habits and provide simple solutions for wellness among young adults.

Before we discuss the action plan map, let us consider the three minds Sigmund Freud described, which we all have.

The conscious mind

The creative mind encompasses our thoughts and awareness.

The preconscious mind

It is where we store information in our memory that we can retrieve at any given time.

The subconscious mind

It is the storage of feelings, emotions, and thoughts that we have little control over, and, generally, most stored feelings are negative.

Negative thoughts can set us back and be discouraging, but the more aware we become of them, the sooner we can redirect them toward positive thinking.

Our thoughts create communication between neurons in the brain, which then trigger emotions. These emotions can be positive or negative. The critical factor is that we all have a powerful, blissful nature. However, we realize this at different stages of our lives, or, as noted earlier, in other seasons. Most young people come to this realization later in their lives.

I admit that I realized this in my late thirties and early forties. I am glad that my adult children have reached this realization much earlier. That is one of the reasons I wanted to write this guidebook: to serve as a catalyst for younger generations to recognize their blissful nature and learn how to tap into it to overcome life's challenges. Another fact I've come to realize is that, regardless of chronological age, there's a youthful energy force that remains untainted by age, which is the impressive nature of humans and our cheerleaders that propel us forward in life. We need to embrace this.

Overcoming Negative Beliefs

Beliefs can be empowering on the one hand and limiting on the other. It is empowering to believe that we are human beings with infinite possibilities and can achieve anything we set our minds to. However, our beliefs about ourselves and our lives are often limiting, which can be disempowering. So, how do we shift our assumptions? First, we can do this by recognizing the nature of our thoughts and questioning their origin. How sure are we of the true nature and reality of our beliefs?

Let Us Delve into Self-Reflection

Reflecting on our thoughts, feelings, and experiences can be a valuable tool in our self-development journey. Journaling offers a structured way to record our thoughts, feelings, and experiences over time. Putting pen to paper (or fingers to keyboard) creates a tangible record of our innermost thoughts and emotions, helping us track patterns, identify triggers, and gain insight into our behavior. When engaging in self-reflection through journaling, honesty and openness with yourself are essential. Allow yourself to explore your thoughts and feelings without judgment or self-censorship.

Embrace vulnerability and authenticity, knowing that genuine growth comes from confronting the uncomfortable truths within ourselves. Self-reflection can benefit us in several ways, supporting our personal development and well-being. It can help us become more attuned to our thoughts, emotions, and behaviors. Sitting quietly with ourselves and asking, "Who am I, and what makes me happy?" can help us make better decisions, set priorities and goals for our lives, and feel more fulfilled. Our emotional intelligence increases when we engage in self-reflection.

For example, every day before going to bed, reflect on the day, recognize and assess one's feelings, and empathize with the feelings of others you encountered. By engaging in this type of self-assessment, one can notice personal growth. It helps identify areas that require improvement. It is a form of self-care and self-expression, and therefore helps reduce stress and promote relaxation. Through this reflective practice, one can begin to unlock one's true potential. Being present in the moment is crucial for our self-awareness. If you feel comfortable, ask a confidant or a mentor for their views on your strengths and weaknesses.

Moreover, we can look more deeply into ourselves to see how we would feel if our old belief that it is not helping us were invalid. What would I think if that thought were not true? How would our lives be without that disempowering belief? We could create new beliefs by first imagining them.

Our imagination can work for us if we direct it to a space or place where we feel safe, relaxed, and happy. Simply put, I want you to understand the power your mind has to shape your thoughts. Acknowledge that, and know you can grant your mind permission to direct itself toward happy thoughts that empower you.

Meditate and Quiet the Mind

People are encouraged to meditate to quiet their minds and find relaxation. Sitting quietly and focusing on your breathing detoxifies the mind of past beliefs, opens it to new, happy feelings and thoughts, and helps achieve a state of mind that supports and encourages change.

First, we need to acknowledge this and own our conscious and unconscious thoughts. Beliefs are assumptions and conclusions drawn from information and experience, whether conscious or unconscious. Based on your beliefs, you tend to perceive the world. Your perception can significantly affect your self-esteem, relationships, and how you present yourself across various aspects of your life, including work, social life, and community involvement. It can also affect your spiritual way of looking at the world and your mental health.

Therefore, if you harbor negative thoughts about yourself due to past experiences and beliefs, it is essential to shift them toward more positive ones to enhance your overall well-being. You can immediately move your thoughts to a level that makes you feel good rather than sad, anxious, or scared.

The way to change is to change how we perceive a situation, such as by raising our consciousness. This way, we can break the cycle of beliefs or memes anchored in our subconscious mind, or the "behind-the-scenes mind." Some thoughts are ideas or ways of thinking that have been imposed on us for generations. We believe them to be true because someone else has mentioned them to us, and they are then recycled back into our minds. So, if they are not valid, these ideas, recycled in our subconscious mind as beliefs, can prevent us from growing from within.

Rob Williams, the originator of Psych-K, has developed a practical, simple way to help people rewrite their beliefs. He explains that perception controls behavior, influences genes, and can even alter both genes and behavior. Beliefs influence perception, and if you can rewrite your beliefs, you can rewrite your perception and, consequently, your genes. I am posing these questions to begin understanding one's beliefs and, therefore, to find ways to seek solutions from within.

Table 1. Questioning Thoughts on The Mind

Questions	Questions on Your Mind					
Why What How When Where Who	Are you happy with yourself?	Do you think highly of yourself?	Do you accept yourself as you are?	Do you believe in yourself?	Do you spend time alone?

You are not alone if you answered no to all or most of these questions. Allow yourself to be in a quiet space. Set aside sufficient time for this practice. Take a moment to consider each question individually. Give yourself time to ask why, what, how, when, where, and who, directing these questions inward. I have learned several techniques to overcome negative thoughts and transform them into positive thoughts and beliefs. Below are simple solutions that can help with this process.

Table 2: **Practice Example to Take Action for Mind Shift**

Questions	Negative Thoughts	Positive Thoughts
• Why do I find it hard to accept myself? • What do I want out of life? • Who is responsible for my happiness? • When did the pattern of the negative beliefs start? • Where do I feel happy and safe? • How do I start a new and improve my life?		

Draw two columns: one for negative thoughts and another for positive thoughts. After some time, review your notes and meditate on them, then see how to shift the energy of negative thoughts into the positive column, turning them into a more positive outcome in your favor. This practice may take different amounts of time for each individual.

Studies on self-esteem have found that many young adults

struggle with low self-esteem and a lack of self-love. Thus, most negative issues stem from not appreciating and loving oneself and from being overly self-critical.

It is disheartening to see young people not appreciate themselves. They love or admire movie stars, athletes, or famous musicians, but if asked to look at themselves in the mirror and say, 'I love you,' how would they feel? Most young adults would cringe at the idea of such an action. The sooner someone begins to accept and love themselves in this very moment, the faster accumulated unhealthy thoughts can dissolve, opening the way for a brighter path.

A straightforward way to shift toward more positive beliefs about yourself is to look in the mirror and speak kindly to yourself. For example, look in the mirror and say, "I love and appreciate myself." It may feel strange at first, but as you continue this practice, it becomes more natural and your self-appreciation increases.

You can consider the root cause of negative thoughts. Is it because we were told we were not good enough at some point in our lives? The starting point for solving life's issues and problems is being kind and loving to yourself. Loving yourself brings self-acceptance and self-awareness, no matter the moment or situation you find yourself in. That realization and acceptance can bring so much powerful energy to fruition. Mentally, you become calmer and more at ease with yourself and the world around you.

Upon reflection, we realize that our best body is our own. Your body is beautifully designed to protect you from harm and to have your back. Simply put, wouldn't it be fair for us to have our bodies back, too? So why not start looking at ourselves through a kinder lens, be more appreciative, and speak with more respect?

I often hear clients, friends, and family say, "I will be happy with myself when I lose this weight, get a better job, or finish my studies," or use similar excuses. The key point to remember is that we only have this moment to appreciate, and it is now. This moment is the present moment. In literature, many philosophers have emphasized the power of the present. When we choose to listen to our inner wisdom, which also points to the power of now, we understand that whatever we look forward to, for example, happiness, must start now. Omar Khayyam said, "Be happy at this moment. This moment is your life."

When viewed scientifically, our cells possess memory and can sense what we say and do to our bodies, as evidenced by the research of Dr. Candice Pert and Robert Williams. You can change your behavior through visualization and affirmation, thereby moving toward a more positive mindset. By "visualization," I mean finding your life purpose and what brings you happiness. It is noted that when we begin to visualize how we can serve humanity with our talent, it brings a sense of purpose and, therefore, more positive thoughts. The power of affirmation lies in meditating on what we desire in our lives, maintaining our thoughts and feelings toward that desire, and affirming it to ourselves, which can bring about positive feelings.

Another practical way to maintain positivity in life is to cultivate gratitude. Being grateful brings high energy into our bodies. A simple proof is that when you are thankful, you cannot be angry at yourself, anyone else, or any situation that arises in life. Of course, we all face different challenges in life. However, the challenges in our lives can be resolved more smoothly when we are thankful. I shared my experiences, some of my adult children's experiences, and what I discovered while researching the health of young adults, hoping it would help the younger generation. In conclusion, I want to reassure you not to be too hard on yourself and to recognize that there are ways to achieve healthier, happier lives by discovering your inner potential.

This guidebook is designed to help you embrace your youth and provide practical solutions to the challenges you face on your life's journey.

Chapter 4

Participatory Resilience Wellness Action Challenge

In this chapter, I have designed a map of action plans you can use to address lifestyle and self-esteem issues and to find practical solutions to problems on your journey toward well-being.

The following are some ways we can use to our advantage to overcome new challenges and develop the resilience we need as we live independently on our journey toward well-being.

Independence and Autonomy

Living away from home can foster a sense of independence and the freedom to make your own decisions and take responsibility. It can contribute to your empowerment and self-efficacy. It can also be a way to face challenges head-on by embracing discomfort. Facing new challenges head-on, even when uncomfortable, builds mental strength and adaptability.

I moved to another country at a young age, and it was tough because I was used to having everything supervised by my parents. Becoming independent was a shock to my system. It was a learning curve, and now I realize it made me stronger. However, there was so much I still did not know and was unfamiliar with that I felt despair and a sense of victimhood at the time. I did not realize that moving away from home provided an opportunity for growth.

Personal Growth and Learning

When I left my home country for the UK, I was fortunate to have two of my sisters already there, who provided me with a sense of security and support. However, I was shy and immature when expressing my opinion on certain matters. I did not know how to be assertive or stand up for myself. I had much to learn about valuing my opinion and appreciating myself. I tended to value other people's views more than my own. Then I would have internal conflicts about why I hadn't stood up for myself in so many situations. After a few decades, I realized that a mindset shift transforms obstacles into stepping stones for personal growth. I realized that exposure to new environments, cultures, and people fosters opportunities for personal growth. It led to increased adaptability, resilience, and a broader perspective on life. I hope young readers can reach these solutions earlier than I did.

Career Opportunities and Building Social Connections

Many of us move away from home for educational and career opportunities. Access to better academic and professional options can enhance a sense of purpose and fulfillment. By living away from home, we have the chance to meet new people and build a diverse social network. Strong connections support emotional well-being, strengthen support systems, and foster a sense of belonging.

I remember joining a language school when I moved to the UK. I enjoyed being part of a group of young adults from different parts of the world who were learning a new language. I certainly had fun laughing at the mistakes I made in the language. It was amusing that, in those days, we didn't have cell phones. When the phone rang, my sisters and I would beg each other to answer it, afraid we wouldn't understand the details of the conversation. At times, I would mix the two languages in one sentence. When someone asked a question, I didn't understand, so I would smile and nod. A sense of humor adds strength to one's character.

Balanced Diet, Nutritional Habits, and Lifestyle Factors

As mentioned earlier, research shows that when we are young, we tend to be exposed to ready-to-eat processed foods. By cooking for ourselves, we can take control of our meals. We can learn to include a variety of foods from all food groups in our diet, including fruits, vegetables, whole grains, lean proteins, healthy fats, seaweed, nuts, seeds, herbs, fermented foods, and spices, while avoiding excessive consumption of processed foods, sugary snacks, and high-fat meals. If you decide to include meat and fish in your diet, you should be more mindful of how the animals were raised and what they were fed, and, above all, be grateful to the animals for providing you with food.

You can also be mindful of water and hydration. Drink enough water throughout the day to stay hydrated. Limit sugary and alcoholic beverages if possible. Avoid alcohol altogether and opt for water, herbal teas, or infused water. Aim for regular, balanced meals by avoiding skipping meals, especially breakfast, which provides essential nutrients and sets the tone for the day. For snacks, choose fruits, nuts, and no-sugar-added yogurt to support healthy eating habits.

I have noticed that people living alone often watch TV or use their mobile devices during mealtime. I would encourage them to be mindful of what they watch, especially if it makes them feel good.

Incorporating regular exercise and adequate sleep into your routine is essential to mental resilience, as it builds coping mechanisms and fosters self-care.

I remember that during my younger years, I was unaware of the importance of mindful eating and how much exercise I needed. However, my childhood diet and lifestyle were mainly Mediterranean and Middle Eastern, with a variety of fruits, vegetables, nuts, seeds, whole grains, beans, and pulses. My mother always prepared homemade meals for us. Those habits laid a solid foundation for my young adulthood. I was very active in sports and was part of the high school volleyball team. In that sense, those habits laid a strong foundation for my independent living.

As for sleep hygiene, our friends would visit us and were used to staying up late. I would say good night to them if I needed to sleep early, after ten o'clock. They would tease me at times, asking, "Are you chicken? Why do you go to bed so early?" I am glad I listen to my body's sleep cues rather than trying to please others.

Relaxation and Meditation

Identify and address sources of stress or friction in your life to maintain mental well-being. Then practice stress-reducing activities, such as meditation and the techniques mentioned earlier. Mindfulness and meditation can help reduce stress and maintain emotional balance. Repeated mindfulness practice enhances your ability to stay calm under pressure. Experiment with different modalities to see which works best for you, whether you listen to classical or uplifting music, breathe, do yoga, or sing. Research indicates that listening to music you enjoy can boost the immune system, alleviate stress, and ultimately improve overall well-being. Once again, I want to emphasize the power of gratitude and how it can shift your perspective and improve your overall well-being. Focus on the positive aspects of life and on what you can control, rather than on what you cannot or have not. I was not introduced to meditation and mindfulness concepts at a young age. However, I knew that going for a walk in nature, laughing with a few friends, listening to a happy song, dancing, or simply visiting a coffee shop or tea house and enjoying scones and tea with family and friends used to lift my spirits.

Social Connections

Maintaining positive social connections with friends, family, and the community benefits overall well-being. Build a support system by sharing experiences and receiving emotional support through a strong network of friends, family, and mentors. Sharing your struggles and seeking advice can provide new perspectives and emotional support.

When I moved to the UK, my sisters and I befriended a few people from the language school and a few more at the college. We were fortunate to find two families in particular. One had two sisters who lived nearby, within walking distance of us. There were times when we felt sad or lonely. We would call our friends, and they would say, "Come over, and I'll put the kettle on." The other family consisted of four sisters and two brothers, with whom we shared many happy times. I still keep in touch with them whenever I visit the UK.

We were each other's support system. Spending time with good friends was enjoyable and straightforward, and it also supported our emotional well-being. I am grateful for their friendship. Additionally, when I lived in Alaska in my early thirties, I often had coffee mornings with friends. At times, everyone would talk, and it seemed we were not listening to what anyone said; we were all waiting for our turn to speak. Everyone wanted to speak up, as I call it, to get it out of their system. Then we would all feel a sense of relief after the coffee morning session. Looking back, I realize those coffee mornings were a form of therapy for us, especially during Alaska's dark winters.

Protecting Your Future: Alcohol, Substance Misuse, and You

The early years of adulthood are dynamic and challenging, marked by new freedoms, new pressures, and the powerful human urge to fit in. Because your brain is still developing, you are especially vulnerable to poor judgment and to the influence of destructive behavior.

This is why mindfulness and clear boundaries are your greatest defense. It is critical to be keenly aware of your alcohol intake—if you choose to drink at all—and to fully commit to avoiding all non-prescribed drug use. The short-term desire to experiment or belong is never worth the long-term impact on your health, future, and mental clarity.

Protecting Your Body

Your body is your most valuable asset and deserves your absolute respect and care. Be intensely mindful of what you put into it.

Alcohol, nicotine, and recreational drugs are not harmless experiments; they are chemicals that compromise your health, clarity, and future.

Never allow yourself to be coerced or pressured into drinking, smoking, or using any substance. Your right to say 'No' is non-negotiable, and prioritizing your well-being is the ultimate sign of self-respect. Protecting your body is the most important decision you make each day.

I am glad to say that I never liked the smell of cigarettes and did not want to be in a room where smoke was in the air. However, back then, smoking in public areas was not restricted, and even on planes, there were designated areas where people would smoke. We were all exposed to smoke either at home or outdoors because there were no strict laws regulating cigarette smoking. Thank goodness it has all changed.

Regular Health Check-ups

When you are young, scheduling regular health check-ups and screenings is not a priority. However, it is an effective way to address any health concerns promptly.

Time Management

Develop practical time-management skills to balance work, studies, and personal life. To reduce stress, prioritize tasks and set realistic goals. Keep a journal and a calendar to track appointments.

I recall working in a hospital back then and how vital my

journal and diary were for tracking my appointments and visits. With today's technology, younger generations can maintain a digital calendar and take notes on their phones or computers much more easily.

Continuous Learning

Engage in lifelong learning and personal development. Pursue hobbies and interests to foster intellectual well-being. Practice critical thinking and decision-making to strengthen your ability to tackle problems. Approach issues methodically to find practical solutions.

Being receptive to discoveries and new findings, realizing that what one believed years ago could be far from the truth after further investigation. Admitting our mistakes and being willing to learn a new way of doing something are steps toward personal growth.

Setting Goals for Lifestyle Habits

In the literature, the acronym SMART is used for goal setting. The acronym for SMART goals stands for Specific, Measurable, Achievable, Relevant, and Time-bound. You can use this framework to set short-term and long-term goals, such as saving money each month and preparing for emergencies. Create a monthly budget that allocates funds for essentials, including rent, groceries, transportation, discretionary spending, emergencies, and medical expenses. Ensuring you have secure housing is crucial for feeling safe.

Maslow's hierarchy of needs lists the requirements, from bottom to top, as physiological (food and clothing), safety (a safe living place and job security), love and belonging needs (friendship), self-esteem, and self-actualization. Self-actualization is at the top of the hierarchy of needs and is achieved only after all the other needs are met. In other words, before we can attend to higher needs, the lower needs in the hierarchy must be met. Therefore, food, shelter, and a safe place to live will bring stability to our lives.

You can also acknowledge that professional advice is available when needed. Free counseling services through social services are available in different cities and, on a larger scale, in many countries.

I remember when we were younger and needed legal advice. There was a Citizen Advisory Bureau, and we approached them several times, receiving help as needed.

Being away from familiar surroundings may lead to feelings of isolation and loneliness, which can negatively affect mental health and overall well-being. Adapting to a new environment, whether in an academic or workplace setting, can be challenging. You may have difficulty adjusting, which can lead to stress and a sense of overwhelm. Being away from family and long-time friends may mean a lack of immediate emotional support.

Establishing a new support system is crucial, and its absence can affect mental health. Your experiences vary, and your well-being while living away from home depends on personal resilience, available support systems, and the living environment. Encouraging a balance between independence and seeking support when needed is crucial for promoting well-being during this transitional phase of life.

As I mentioned earlier, I had to adjust my budget for food and expenses. For example, my sisters and I would grocery shop for the week and set aside a portion of fruit and vegetables for each of us to eat throughout the week. Having a food shopping list ensured I bought the necessary items. Having a few good friends to socialize with wherever I lived was very helpful.

I shall explore food and lifestyle, and how to create desirable habits that benefit you. These healthy habits and lifestyle factors contribute to well-being, promoting physical, mental, and emotional health. It's essential to recognize that well-being is a holistic concept and that gradual, sustainable changes can positively impact various aspects of life.

The Map of Participatory Wellness Action Plan

As mentioned earlier, our perceptions of a problem or an issue differ. Your way of thinking, beliefs, culture, and environment can influence perception. For example, when examining nutrition and lifestyle habits, we can see that individuals' nutritional practices and physical activity levels are influenced by their abilities, thinking, culture, and environmental factors. When assessing a situation, we must consider how the issue was addressed in the past and how we would like to address it now and in the future.

Diagram1. The participatory cycle of wellness change

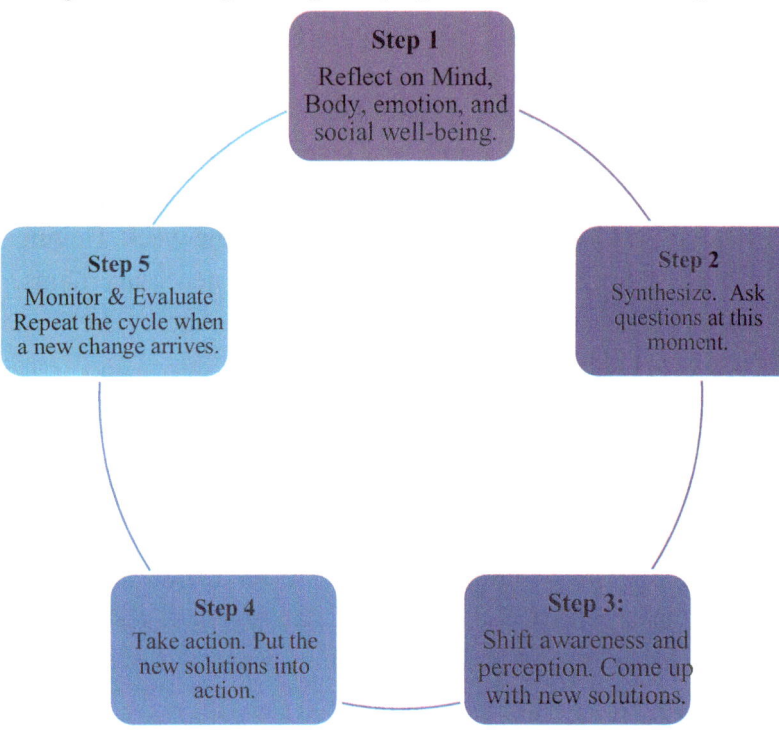

The participatory cycle of wellness change can help address wellness issues, expand our consciousness, and acquire new knowledge.

Reflect, synthesize, shift awareness and perception, take action, monitor the change, and repeat this cycle. One can reflect on and synthesize a situation or problem in the present moment. This change cycle involves developing a new solution or perspective on an issue, shifting one's awareness and perception of the situation or problem from the past to the present, taking action, and designing a strategic solution. For example, if the point of reference is wellness, you can record their experiences managing diet- and lifestyle-related problems, including nutritional habits, exercise routines, and social aspects. You can understand what has worked for you in the past, the steps you are taking now, and how you will continue to do so in the future. Identify successful ways to overcome barriers by asking the questions I mentioned earlier and directing them at yourself. Then think and meditate on ways to overcome obstacles related to physical activity, behavior, and food choices. Monitor and record the change cycle every time an issue arises.

Allocate a timeframe for the process of continual reflection, problem synthesis, shifts in awareness and perception, taking action, and monitoring and evaluation. This challenge demonstrates that when you are the primary stakeholders in developing and implementing systems to address issues such as unhealthy eating habits and low physical activity, the outcomes can be more sustainable.

You can assess your food choices, learn practical ways to improve your eating habits, and make emotional and behavioral changes to achieve healthier weight-related behaviors. This challenge could help you become more independent and encourage you to develop a strategic plan to tackle barriers to your wellness by being more attuned to the physical, emotional, mental, and social aspects of your life.

Practical Strategies for Building Resilience

Writing about your experiences and emotions can help you process them effectively and track your progress. Learning to say no and setting boundaries to protect your time and energy helps prevent burnout and keeps you focused on your priorities. You become more resilient by challenging yourself and reframing negative thoughts into more positive or realistic ones. Acknowledging and celebrating your achievements, no matter how small, reinforces positive behavior and builds momentum. Resilient individuals experience lower levels of anxiety and depression and are better equipped to handle life's ups and downs.

Building resilience is an ongoing process that involves facing challenges, developing coping strategies, and maintaining a positive attitude. Strong coping skills and a positive mindset contribute to healthier, more fulfilling relationships. By integrating these strategies into your daily life, you can empower yourself to overcome obstacles and thrive in the face of adversity. You can help each other by sharing ideas that have worked for you to develop a healthier lifestyle, encouraging physical activity, reducing stress, and detoxifying the mind and emotions. Dr. Deepak Chopra notes that our awareness shifts when we acquire new knowledge.

Through my life experiences, I have learned that the hardships I endured in my youth helped shape my patience and resilience. I remember wishing I had better options at certain times in my life and wondering how to achieve them. However, as life passed, I realized that things happened at the right time, and I wish to pass this message on to you.

Chapter 5
Recipes For a Wellness Journey

In previous chapters, I assessed risk factors and benefactors for your wellness journey. I also examined how you can improve your life by accepting and appreciating yourself at any moment. I included a participatory action plan map to guide your wellness journey. In this chapter, I have included vegetarian recipes with vegan options to support your wellness journey. These recipes are designed to incorporate more fruits, vegetables, nuts, seeds, herbs, and spices into your diet. Preparing homemade meals with a variety of vegetarian options can help you take control of your dietary choices and make informed decisions about your health. These recipes are practical, simple, quick, economical, plant-rich, and nutrient-dense, offering a wealth of fiber, vitamins, minerals, polyphenols, and antioxidants. Vegetarian meals can support the immune system and boost energy levels.

Furthermore, including vegetarian and vegan options can have heart health benefits. A plant-rich diet can aid weight management by promoting a healthier gut microbiome and better digestion. Fruits, vegetables, whole grains, and legumes are rich in fiber and support the digestive system. Often, people wonder whether a vegetarian diet provides enough calcium and protein. Green, leafy vegetables, nuts and seeds, beans and lentils, fermented soy products, sea vegetables, and algae such as spirulina are good sources of calcium, protein, vitamins, and minerals.

Plant-rich foods help protect against chronic diseases, including diabetes, cancer, and obesity. Because of their fiber and complex carbohydrate content, whole foods can help stabilize blood sugar levels. Vegetarian meals can add variety to one's diet by using a variety of fruits, vegetables, nuts, seeds, herbs, and spices. From a budget perspective, plant-rich foods are more economical.

Food and mood are strongly linked; plants can positively affect mood and, in turn, contribute to improved mental health. Developing healthy eating habits from a young age can help reduce the risk of chronic diseases as one ages.

One important note is to ensure that B12, Vitamin D, and omega-3 fatty acids are at optimal levels and to consult your physician about appropriate supplementation.

If you eat animal-based foods, be mindful of portion size, the animal's treatment, and the feed used. Above all, be grateful to animals and plants for the food and nourishment they provide. The recipes are either oil-free or cooked with high-quality, extra-virgin olive oil, which offers numerous benefits. Depending on one's medical condition, it is recommended to consult a general practitioner and a dietitian for personalized advice. This information is educational and should not replace one's doctor's recommendation.

Recipes

Olives And Oil Extracted from Olives

Olives and oil extracted from olives are rich in monounsaturated fats, particularly oleic acid. Replacing saturated and trans fats with monounsaturated fats can help lower blood pressure and reduce the risk of heart disease. Olive oil contains antioxidants, vitamin E, and phenolic compounds, such as oleuropein, hydroxytyrosol, and tyrosol. These antioxidants help protect cells from oxidative stress and the inflammation associated with chronic diseases, such as heart disease and cancer. The phenolic compounds in olive oil have anti-inflammatory properties. Regular consumption of olives and olive oil may reduce inflammation, potentially lowering the risk of chronic inflammatory diseases. Consuming olives, olive oil, and olive polyphenols can benefit bone health. Some studies suggest that the monounsaturated fats in olive oil may protect the brain and reduce the risk of cognitive decline and neurodegenerative diseases, such as Alzheimer's. Although calorie-dense, olive oil can still be an integral part of a healthy diet. Its monounsaturated fats can promote satiety and reduce overall calorie intake when used in moderation, potentially aiding in weight management. Olives may aid digestion by stimulating the gallbladder to release bile, which helps break down fats. Some studies suggest that olive oil's antioxidants and anti-inflammatory compounds may help reduce the risk of certain cancers, particularly those of the breast, colon, and prostate. Olive oil is used in skincare and hair care products due to its moisturizing and nourishing properties. When applied topically, it can help hydrate the skin and hair.

Some evidence suggests that olives and high-quality olive oil, especially when consumed as part of a Mediterranean diet, support better bone health and a lower risk of osteoporosis. The Mediterranean diet, which features olive oil as a staple, has been linked to increased longevity and a lower risk of age-related diseases.

Vegan Egg Alternative

Tofu and tempeh are versatile plant-based protein sources made from soybeans. Choose organic and fermented varieties if possible. They have a protein content similar to eggs and can be used in various dishes, such as scrambles and quiches, or as a substitute in baking. Protein content ranges from 10 to 20 grams per 3.5 ounces (100 grams), depending on the type. They also provide essential amino acids, iron, calcium, and other minerals. Tempeh is also a protein-rich food, containing about 19 grams per 3.5 ounces (100 grams). It's high in fiber, vitamins, and minerals, including manganese, phosphorus, and magnesium. Tempeh also contains probiotics, which are beneficial for gut health.

Edamame: Young soybeans, which can be boiled or

steamed, are a good source of protein.

Chickpea Flour (also known as gram flour) is high in protein and can be used to make chickpea omelets or savory pancakes. Its texture and taste resemble those of eggs. One can add herbs and spices to enhance the dish's flavor and antioxidant content.

Legume Scramble

Mashed or blended legumes, such as lentils or chickpeas, can be seasoned and cooked to create a texture similar to scrambled eggs. Mashed legumes are an alternative to eggs. Chickpea flour is high in protein, with about 20 grams per one cup (92 grams). It's also a good source of fiber, iron, folate, and other nutrients. Chickpeas are used in the food industry to make bread, sandwiches, soups, pasta, crackers, cakes, beverages, mayonnaise-like dressings, and gluten-free pasta, among other food products. Legumes, such as lentils and chickpeas, are rich in protein, fiber, vitamins, and minerals. Legume scrambles can provide about 15-20 grams of protein per serving (one cup, cooked), depending on the type and preparation method. They also offer complex carbohydrates and various micronutrients.

Nutritional Yeast

It has a cheesy flavor and is often used to add a savory taste to plant-based dishes. It's a good source of B vitamins, protein, and fiber, and it can be sprinkled on tofu scrambles or other plant-based dishes or used as part of a dish's seasoning. Start with a small amount and develop a taste for it. Nutritional yeast contains approximately 8 grams of protein per 1/4 cup (60 grams). It's an excellent source of B vitamins, particularly B12, in plant-based diets. Nutritional yeast also adds a savory flavor to dishes and can enhance their nutritional profile.

Herbal Cutlet Squares (Gluten-Free)

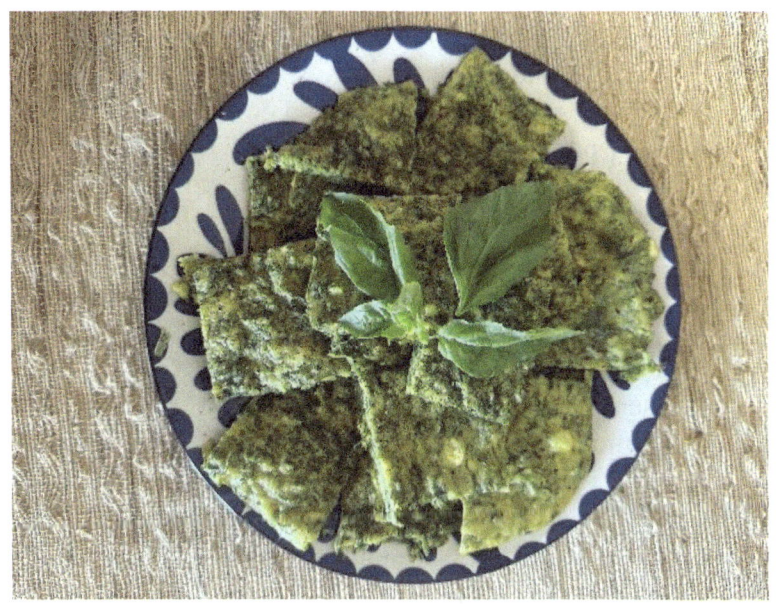

Preparation time: 30 minutes
Cooking time: 20 minutes
Serving: 4

Ingredients:
- ✓ 4 organic, free-range, pasture-raised eggs (vegan option below), 200-240g (7-8.5 oz.)
- ✓ 2 organic medium-sized potatoes, 300-400g (10.5-14 oz.)
- ✓ 1 medium-sized onion (150-200 g) or one teaspoon or 5 g onion powder
- ✓ ½ teaspoon turmeric, 2.5g (0.05 oz.)
- ✓ ½ teaspoon curry powder, 2.5g (0.05 oz.)
- ✓ 1 cup of chopped parsley, cilantro, and dill, 30-40g (1-1.5 oz.)
- ✓ 2 cloves of garlic, chopped, 10-15g (0.3-0.5 oz.)
- ✓ ½ cup rice flour or chickpea flour, 60-70g (2-2.5 oz.)
- ✓ ¼ cup of olive oil, 60g (2 oz.)
- ✓ Salt and pepper to taste, 5-10g (0.2-0.4 oz.)
- ✓ 1 serrano pepper, 15-20g (0.5-0.7 oz.)
- ✓ 1 lemon (optional)

Recipe:
1. Boil the potatoes in a small pan. Allow them to cool, remove the skin, and mash them with a potato masher or a fork.
2. Mix the eggs in a Pyrex dish with chopped herbs, spices, onion, and garlic.
3. Add the mashed potatoes and the rice flour or chickpea flour to the mixture and mix well.
4. Place parchment paper and olive oil in an oven tray.
5. Then pour the whole mixture into the oven tray.
6. Cook in the oven at 350°F for eighteen minutes.
7. Cut the cutlet into square shapes.

8. Serve with salad.

Nutritional Values of an Egg

Calories: 72 kcal
Protein: 6.3 grams
Fat: 4.8 grams
Saturated Fat: 1.6 grams
Monounsaturated Fat: 2 grams
Polyunsaturated Fat: 0.7 grams
Carbohydrates: 0.6 grams

Eggs are renowned for their high-quality protein, which provides all the essential amino acids needed for human health. They are also rich in vitamins and minerals, especially vitamin B12, choline, and selenium. Additionally, eggs are a good source of healthy fats, including monounsaturated and polyunsaturated fats, and they contain essential nutrients for eye health, such as lutein and zeaxanthin. The nutrient content of eggs can vary slightly based on factors such as egg size, the chicken's diet, the method of raising (e.g., pasture-raised), and the method of preparation (e.g., boiling, frying, scrambling). Eggs are versatile and nutritious and can be part of a balanced diet.

The Vegan Option

Follow the same recipe, but replace the eggs with one cup of chickpea flour or one can of organic chickpeas. Mash the chickpeas with the potatoes, then mix with herbs and spices, rice flour, one tablespoon of nutritional yeast, and olive oil. Pour the mixture into the oven tray. Bake at 350°F for eighteen minutes. Cut the cutlet into square shapes. Serve with salad and a slice of homemade bread.

Total Nutritional Values of the Herbal Cutlet Squares

	Vegan option
Total calories: 1650 Kcal	1700Kcal
Total protein: 45 g	50 g
Total carbohydrates: 117g	155 g
Total Fat: 115 g	100 g
Total fiber: 15 g	28 g

Spicy Herbal Scrambled Eggs

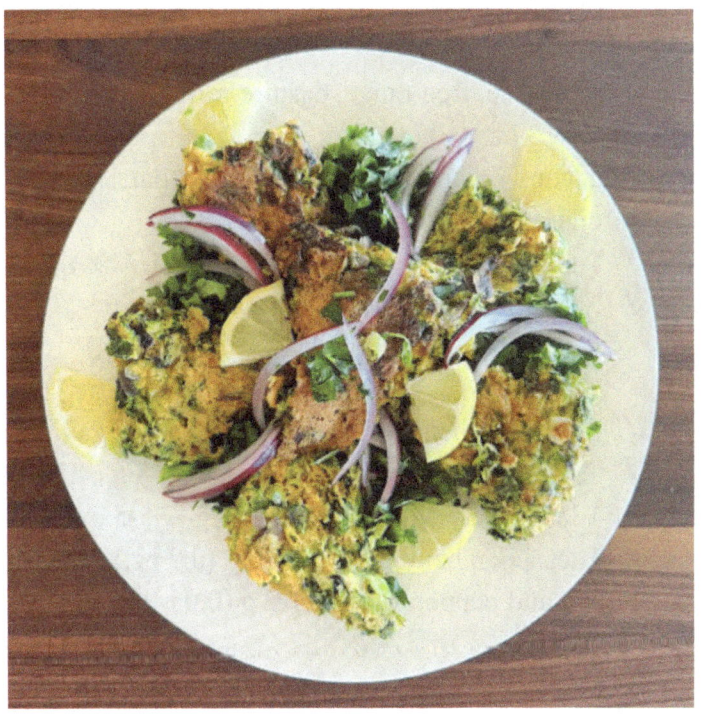

Preparation Time: 30-40 minutes
Cooking Time: 20-30 minutes
Portion Size: 4

Ingredients:

- ✔ 4 organic, free-range, pasture-raised eggs. 200-240 g (7-8.5 oz.)
- ✔ 2 cups of chopped mixed herbs (parsley, dill, and cilantro) 60-80 g (2-2.5 oz.)
- ✔ 1 medium-sized onion, 150-200 g (5-7 oz.)
- ✔ ½ teaspoon turmeric, 2.5 g (0.05 oz.)
- ✔ ½ teaspoon curry powder, 2.5 g (0.05 oz.)
- ✔ ½ teaspoon cayenne pepper, 2.5 g (0.05 oz.)
- ✔ 2 tablespoons good quality olive oil, 30 g (1 oz.)
- ✔ ½ tablespoon non-GMO cornstarch, 8 g (0.3 oz.)
- ✔ 1 leek finely chopped, 100-150 g (3.5-5 oz.)
- ✔ 1 teaspoon baking powder, 5 g (0.2 oz.)
- ✔ salt and pepper to taste, 1-2 g (0.05-0.07 oz.)

Recipe:

1. Using a spoon, mix the eggs, herbs, spices, cornstarch, and baking powder in a medium Pyrex dish, incorporating air into the mixture.
2. In a medium-sized frying pan, heat olive oil over low heat.
3. Add the chopped leek first and allow it to soften. Then add the egg mixture to the frying pan.
4. Cook on a low to medium flame.
5. Place a lid on the frying pan to improve heat distribution.

6. Cook for 15 minutes, then set the mixture aside and divide it into four segments.
7. One can serve this dish with two slices of organic sourdough toast and a salad.

For the vegan option, follow the same recipe, but replace the eggs with one cup of chickpea flour or one can of organic chickpeas. Mix the chickpeas with the herbs and spices, rice flour, one tablespoon of nutritional yeast, and olive oil.

Total Nutritional Values of the Herbal Spicy Scrambled Eggs

	Vegan option
Total calories: 820 Kcal	1000 Kcal
Total protein: 38g	30.5 g
Total carbohydrates: 45 g	105 g
Total Fat: 63 g	55 g
Total fiber: 10.5g	22g

Hazelnuts, Pumpkin seeds, and Herbal Tempeh Salad

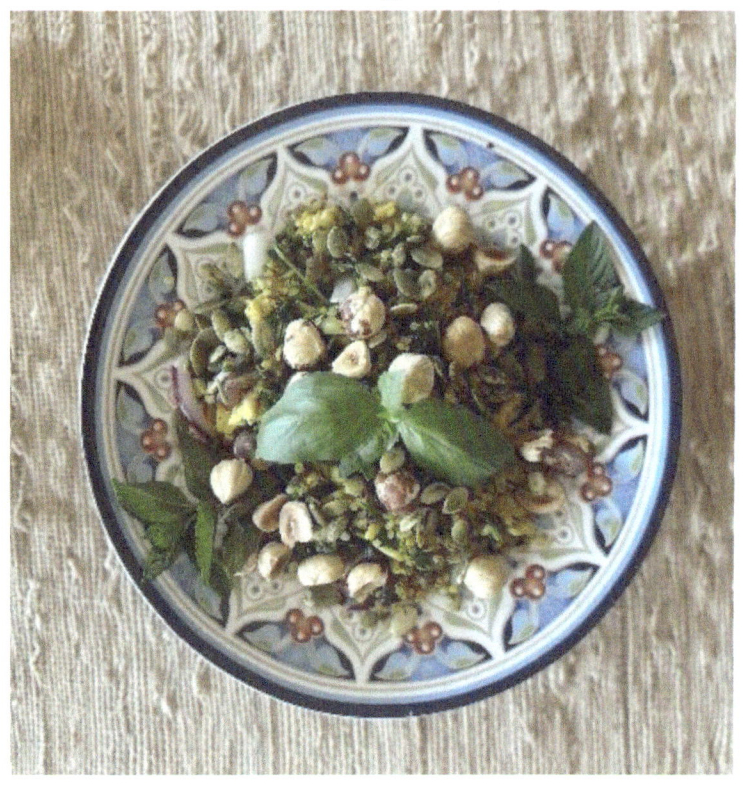

Cooking Time: 20-30 minutes

Preparation Time: 30-40 minutes

Serves: 4

Replace four eggs with one cup of cooked lentils or quinoa and 3 oz of tempeh. Use one cup of cooked lentils or quinoa and 200 g (7 oz) of tempeh, and follow the above recipe, substituting the eggs with these ingredients. Cook the quinoa or lentils in water for 15-30 minutes until tender but not mushy. Drain any excess liquid before using. Adding pumpkin seeds and hazelnuts to the dish increases protein content, is high in zinc and vitamin E, and adds extra flavor.

Total Nutritional Values of Tempeh salad with Eggs	Vegan Option
Total Calories: 594 Kcal	Calories: 620 Kcal
Total Protein: 25g	Protein: 21.5g
Total Fat: 48g	Total Fat: 29g
Total Carbohydrates: 19g	Total Carbohydrates: 75g
Total Fiber: 4g	Fiber: 20.5g

As noted earlier, eggs are a good source of protein, vitamins, and minerals, including vitamins A, D, B12, selenium, and choline. Parsley, cilantro, dill, and leeks are rich in vitamins A, C, and K, as well as various minerals. This dish provides fiber from the vegetables and herbs. The spices have anti-inflammatory and antioxidant properties.

Vegan Option: Herbs, spices, pumpkin seeds, hazelnuts, lentils, quinoa, and soybeans (such as tempeh or tofu) are high in protein and antioxidants, making them a great alternative for vegetarians and vegans.

Lentils and soybeans are rich in dietary fiber, which supports digestive health and helps regulate blood sugar. They are also excellent sources of essential minerals, including iron, magnesium, potassium, and zinc, all of which play vital roles in maintaining normal bodily functions.

Lentils, in particular, are a valuable source of B-complex vitamins. Per 100 g of cooked lentils, they provide approximately:
- Vitamin B1 (Thiamine): 0.41 mg
- Vitamin B2 (Riboflavin): 0.21 mg
- Vitamin B3 (Niacin): 2.1 mg
- Vitamin B5 (Pantothenic Acid): 0.5 mg
- Vitamin B6 (Pyridoxine): 0.5 mg
- Folate (Vitamin B9): 181 mcg

These nutrients contribute to energy metabolism, nervous system function, and overall health.

Spicy Scrambled Tempeh Wrap with Quinoa Bread

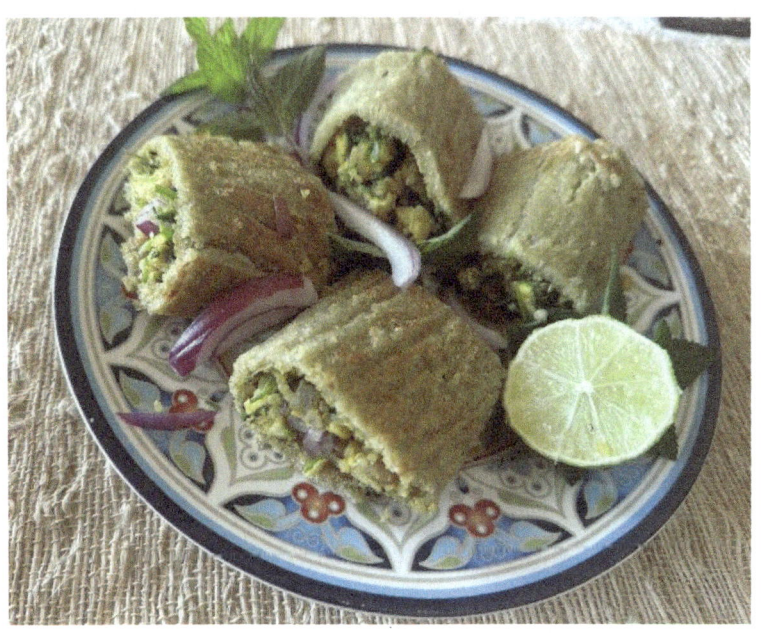

Preparation Time: 20-30 minutes (mainly for washing and chopping herbs and cooking quinoa)
Cooking Time: 20 minutes for quinoa bread and 20 minutes for the scrambled Tempeh recipe
Serves: 4

Ingredients:
- ✓ ½ cup chopped Tempeh or 4 ounces or 112g
- ✓ ½ cup cooked quinoa or 4 ounces and 112g
- ✓ 2 cups of chopped mixed herbs (parsley, dill, and cilantro), 60-80g (2-2.5oz.)
- ✓ 1 medium-sized onion, 150-200g (5-7oz.)
- ✓ ½ teaspoon turmeric, 2.5g (0.05oz.)
- ✓ ½ teaspoon curry powder, 2.5g (0.05oz.)
- ✓ ½ teaspoon cayenne pepper, 2.5g (0.05oz.)
- ✓ 2 tablespoons good quality olive oil, 30g (1 oz.)
- ✓ ½ tablespoon non-GMO cornstarch, 8g (0.3 oz.)
- ✓ 1 leek finely chopped, 100-150g (3.5-5 oz.)
- ✓ 1 teaspoon baking powder, 5g (0.2 oz.)
- ✓ salt and pepper to taste, 1-2g (0.05-0.07oz.)

*Quinoa Bread:
- ✓ 1 cup cooked quinoa or 8 oz. or 225g
- ✓ 1 cup gluten-free flour or 8 oz. or 225g
- ✓ 1 tablespoon olive oil on parchment or ½ oz. or 15g
- ✓ 1 teaspoon baking powder or 5 grams or 0.6 oz.
- ✓ Salt to taste
- ✓ 2 cups of water or 8 oz. or 225g (make adjustments based on your dough)

Recipe:
1. Add the quinoa, gluten-free flour, water, baking powder, and salt to a food processor. Process until the mixture is smooth.

2. Next, add a small amount of olive oil to the parchment paper, then pour the mixture onto the baking sheet lined with it.
3. Preheat the oven to 375°F (190°C). Bake for 20-25 minutes, or until golden brown. Allow to cool.
4. In a large skillet, heat the olive oil over medium heat. Add the diced onion and leek and sauté until they soften.
5. Stir in the chopped tempeh and cook for five minutes.
6. Then add the remaining herbs, cooked quinoa, turmeric, curry powder, cayenne pepper, and mixed herbs. Stir well to combine.
7. In a small bowl, combine cornstarch and water to form a paste. Then, add the paste to the skillet and season with salt and pepper to taste.
8. Assemble the wrap:
    a. Spoon the spicy scrambled tempeh mixture onto quinoa bread.
    b. Fold the bread to create a wrap. Serve warm.

Total Nutritional Values of Scrambled Tempeh Wrap with Quinoa Bread

Calories: 698 Kcal
Protein: 29g
Carbohydrates: 70g
Fat: 50g
Fiber: 14g

Egg Salad With Green Olives

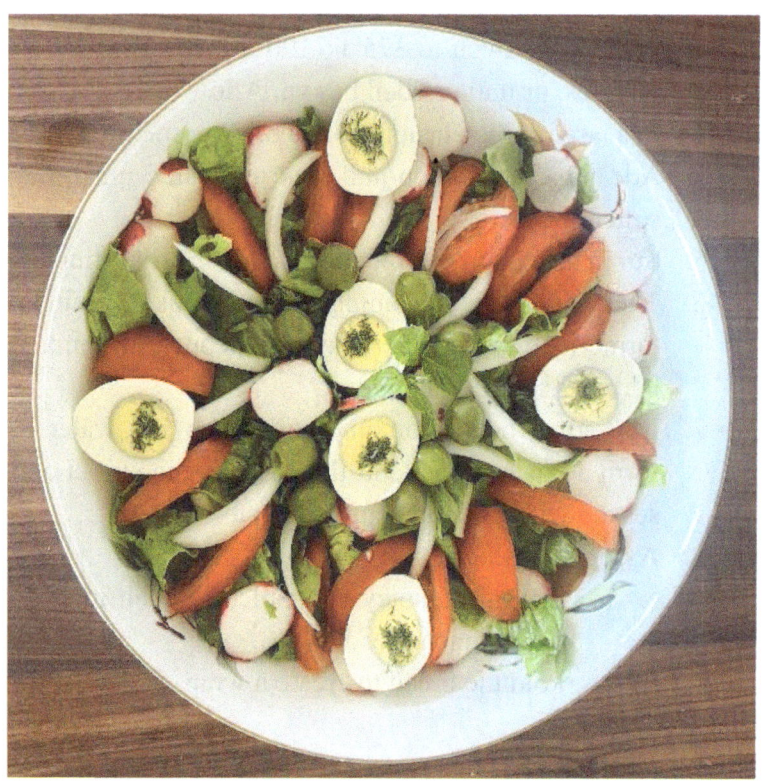

Preparation Time: 20-30 minutes
(Mainly for washing and chopping vegetables, and boiling eggs)
Cooking Time: 15 minutes to boil the eggs.
Vegan option: Replace eggs with cooked organic chickpeas.
Serves: 4

Ingredients:
- ✓ 1 whole organic romaine lettuce, washed, 300-400g (10.5-14oz)
- ✓ 1 medium-sized onion, 150-200g (5-7 oz.)
- ✓ 2 medium-sized tomatoes, 300-400g (10.5-14 oz.)
- ✓ ½ English cucumber, 150-200g (5-7 oz.)
- ✓ 10 olives pitted and chopped, 50-75g (1.8-2.6 oz.)
- ✓ 4 radishes diced, 50-75g (1.8-2.6 oz.)
- ✓ 3 boiled organic eggs, diced into four segments, 200-240g (7-8.5 oz.)
- ✓ 1 teaspoon mustard, 5g (0.2 oz.)
- ✓ 1 tablespoon good quality olive oil, 15g (0.5 oz.)
- ✓ 1 whole lemon juice, 30-60 ml (1-2 Fl oz.)
- ✓ salt and pepper, 1-2 g (0.05-0.07oz.)

Recipe:
1. Wash all the vegetables for the salad, then drain the water in a colander or through a centrifugal water extractor.
2. Chop the salad into pieces to your desired size.
3. Boil the eggs in hot water for 10-15 minutes.
4. Arrange all the ingredients in a salad bowl.
5. Mix mustard, good-quality olive oil, lemon juice, salt, and pepper.
6. Pour over the salad before serving.

Vegetarian Alternative Salad with Chickpeas, Avocado, and decorated with Broccoli Sprouts (The Vegan Option)

Replace the boiled eggs with protein-rich vegan alternatives such as chickpeas. Use one cup of cooked chickpeas or quinoa, one teaspoon of nutritional yeast, and avocado slices. Alternatively, roast the chickpeas in the oven to make them crunchy. You can also use firm tofu, chopped or crumbled, or diced or crumbled tempeh. Mix all the salad ingredients with the dressing.

The Nutritional Values for Egg Salad and Vegan Alternative:

Total calories: 466 Kcal	**Total** Calories: 632 Kcal
Total protein: 21g	**Total** Protein: 32g
Total carbohydrates: 26.5g.	**Total** carbohydrates: 71g
Total fat: 32g	**Total** fat: 34g
Total fiber: 5g	**Total** fiber: 16 g

Eggs, chickpeas, and quinoa are good sources of protein. Onions provide vitamin C, B6 (Pyridoxine), B9 (Folate), potassium, and small amounts of other vitamins and minerals. Tomatoes are rich in vitamins C and A and are a good source of the antioxidant lycopene. Cucumbers are a good source of vitamin K and provide small amounts of vitamin C, potassium, and other nutrients. They are also high in water. Olives are a rich source of vitamin E, iron, copper, calcium, and other essential nutrients. They are also a source of healthy monounsaturated fats.

Vegetable Omelet

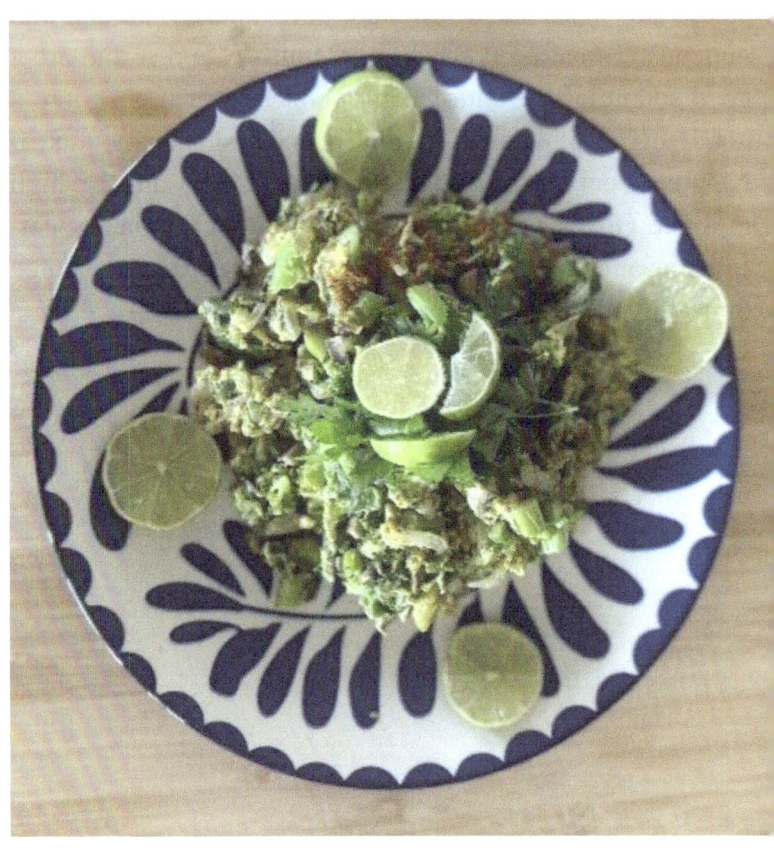

Preparation Time: 15 minutes
Cooking Time: 20 minutes
Serves: 4

Ingredients:
- ✓ 4 organic, free-range, pasture-raised eggs (200g or 7 oz. total)
- ✓ 3 medium-sized organic tomatoes, diced (400g or 14 oz.)
- ✓ 1 medium-sized onion, chopped (150g or 5.3 oz.)
- ✓ ½ teaspoon turmeric (2.5g or 0.05oz.)
- ✓ ½ teaspoon curry powder (2.5g or 0.05oz.)
- ✓ 4 stalks of asparagus, chopped (200g or 7oz.)
- ✓ 4 stalks of celery, chopped (200g or 7oz.)
- ✓ ½ cup chopped parsley (15g or 0.5oz.)
- ✓ 1 tablespoon non-GMO starch (or arrowroot starch, 8g or 0.3oz.)
- ✓ 2 tablespoons good quality olive oil (30g or 1 oz.)
- ✓ salt and pepper to taste 1-2g (0.05-0.07oz.)

Recipe:
1. Mix the eggs, cornstarch, and spices thoroughly in a large bowl.
2. In a pan over low heat, add some good-quality olive oil, then add the chopped vegetables and cook for 5 minutes.
3. Add the egg mixture and spices to the vegetables, then cook for 15 minutes over a low flame.
4. The omelet can be served alone or with a salad and organic sourdough toast.

Vegan Option:
1. Cook one cup of the red lentils in a medium-sized pan with three cups of water.
2. Drain any remaining water after the dish is fully cooked, about 20 minutes over a medium flame. Season with salt and pepper to taste.
3. Mix the cooked lentils with a tablespoon of water and the non-GMO starch (such as cornstarch or arrowroot starch) until the mixture forms a thick, paste-like consistency. Use this lentil mixture as a substitute for eggs in the recipe, following the exact cooking instructions for the vegetables.

Total Nutritional Values of Vegetable Omelet Recipe	**Vegan Option**
Total Calories: 693 Kcal	Total Calories 677 Kcal
Total Protein: 32g	Total Protein: 30.3g
Total Carbohydrates: 40g	Total Carbohydrates: 94.2g
Total Fat: 48g	Total Fat: 29.6g
Total Fiber: 10.5g	Total Fiber: 30.1g

In the previous pages, I explained the nutritional value of the egg. Other ingredients, such as tomatoes, are good sources of vitamins C, K, and folate. Tomatoes also provide minerals like potassium and small amounts of manganese. Onions contain vitamins C and B6 (Pyridoxine), minerals such as potassium, and small amounts of manganese and copper.

Spices such as turmeric contain beneficial compounds, including curcumin, which is known for its potential health benefits. Curry powder is a blend of multiple spices; its nutritional content can vary. Depending on its ingredients, it may contain small amounts of vitamins and minerals. Asparagus and celery are good sources of vitamin K and provide vitamins A, C, and folate. They also contain minerals such as potassium, along with small amounts of iron, manganese, magnesium, and calcium. Chopped parsley is rich in vitamin K and provides vitamins A and C. It contains minerals such as potassium, along with small amounts of calcium and iron. As I explained earlier, olive oil is a source of healthy monounsaturated fats. It contains small amounts of vitamins E and K. Please note that the specific content of vitamins and minerals can vary depending on factors such as the variety and freshness of the ingredients.

Lemon Zest Quinoa Salad

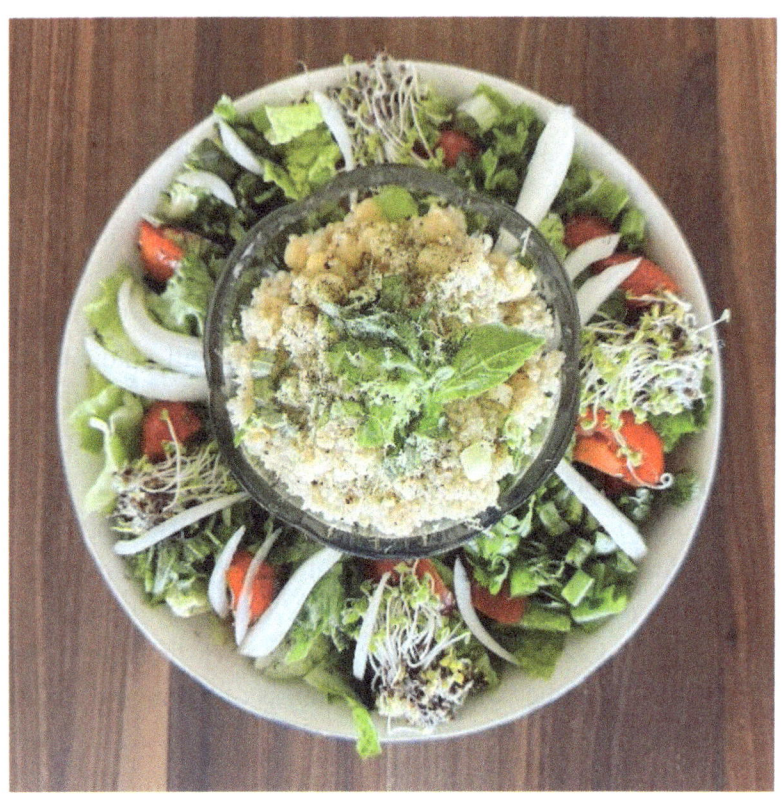

Preparation Time: 15 minutes
Cooking Time: 15-20 minutes
Serves: Serves 4

Ingredients:
- ✓ 1 cup of quinoa (185g or 6.5oz.)
- ✓ 4 green onions or scallions, washed and chopped (60g or 2oz.)
- ✓ 1 large organic Romaine lettuce
- ✓ 1 cup of cooked organic chickpeas (170g or 6oz.)
- ✓ 1 teaspoon mustard (5g or 0.2oz.)
- ✓ 2 medium-sized tomatoes (400g or 14oz.)
- ✓ 2 tablespoons good quality olive oil (30g or 1 oz.)
- ✓ Juice of 1 whole lemon (three tablespoons or 45g or 1.5oz.)
- ✓ ½ teaspoon lemon zest (1g or 0.03oz.)
- ✓ 1 medium-sized onion, chopped (150g or 5.3oz.)
- ✓ 2 tablespoons broccoli sprouts or any other vegetable sprouts available (10g or 0.35oz.)
- ✓ Pinch of organic herbs for decoration
- ✓ Salt and pepper to taste

Recipe:
1. In a small pan, cook the quinoa for 15 minutes, or until the grains are translucent and tender. Pour off any remaining water.
2. Add the cooked quinoa and cooked chickpeas to a large mixing bowl.
3. Add the remaining ingredients, including the olive oil and lemon as a dressing, and incorporate them.

4. This salad can be served on its own or paired with another dish.
5. Decorate with some mixed herbs.

Total Nutritional Values of Lemon Zest Quinoa Salad

Total Calories: 970 Kcal
Total Carbohydrates: 120g
Total Fat: 34.6g
Total Protein: 35g
Total fiber: 35 g

Herbs such as parsley, basil, and dill are rich in polyphenols. Romaine lettuce contains vitamins A, B, C, and K, as well as minerals such as calcium, iron, magnesium, potassium, phosphorus, and sodium. Green onions, also known as scallions, are good sources of vitamins A and K. Chickpeas provide vitamins such as B6 (Pyridoxine), folate, and traces of other B vitamins. Chickpeas are good sources of minerals, including iron, magnesium, phosphorus, and zinc. Avocados contain vitamins such as K, E, and C, as well as various B vitamins. They contain potassium, magnesium, fiber, and trace amounts of other minerals. Lemon juice is a good source of vitamin C. Broccoli sprouts are rich in vitamins C and K. Quinoa contains B vitamins (B1, B2, B3, B6), vitamin E, and minerals such as magnesium, phosphorus, potassium, and iron.

Mom's Hearty Soup

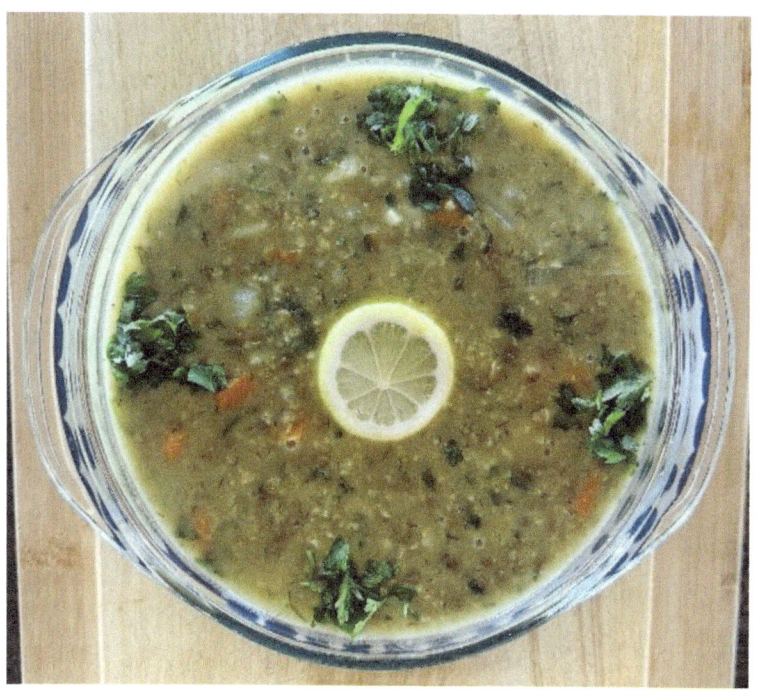

Preparation Time:30 minutes
Cooking Time: 60-75 minutes
Serves: 6

Ingredients:
- ✓ 1 cup organic steel-cut oats (170g or 6 oz.)
- ✓ 1 cup green lentils (200g or 7oz.)
- ✓ ½ cup parsnips, chopped into small pieces (70g or 2.5 oz.)
- ✓ ½ cup chopped onion (70g or 2.5 oz.)
- ✓ ½ cup carrots, cut into small pieces (70g or 2.5 oz.)
- ✓ ½ cup sweet potatoes, cut into small pieces (70g or 2.5 oz.)
- ✓ 1 cup mixed herbs (chopped parsley, dill, coriander) (30g or 1 oz.)
- ✓ 1 teaspoon turmeric (3g or 0.1oz.)
- ✓ 1 teaspoon curry powder (3g or 0.1oz.)
- ✓ 1 chopped Serrano chili, optional
- ✓ 1 teaspoon paprika (3g or 0.1oz.)
- ✓ Salt and pepper to taste
- ✓ 10 cups of water (2.4L or 80 oz.)

Recipe:
1. Soak the lentils for at least an hour.
2. Cook the lentils in a pressure cooker for 20 minutes with four cups of water.
3. Then, in a large pan, add the oats, cooked lentils, and chopped vegetables, along with four cups of water.
4. Cook over medium heat for 15 to 20 minutes.
5. Add the spices to the mixture and adjust the water as needed to reach the desired thickness.
6. Once all the ingredients are fully cooked, serve it on its own or with a slice of organic sourdough toast.

Total Nutritional Values of Mom's Hearty Soup

Total Calories: 738 Kcal
Total Protein: 39g
Total Carbohydrates: 119g
Total Fat: 5g
Total Dietary Fiber: 30g

Parsnips provide vitamins C, K, and folate, along with minerals such as potassium, magnesium, and phosphorus. Onions provide vitamins C, B6 (pyridoxine), and B9 (folate), along with minerals such as potassium, phosphorus, and magnesium. Carrots provide vitamins A (as beta-carotene), K, and C, along with minerals such as potassium, phosphorus, and magnesium. Sweet potatoes contain vitamins A (as beta-carotene), C, and B6 (pyridoxine), along with minerals such as potassium, magnesium, and manganese. Mixed herbs (one cup, including parsley, dill, and coriander) provide vitamins K, C, and folate, along with minerals such as calcium, iron, and magnesium. Serrano chili delivers vitamins C and A. Capsaicin in chili is responsible for the heat. This recipe is a good source of fiber and is low in fat. Turmeric contains curcumin, as indicated earlier, which is known for its potential health benefits. Paprika includes some vitamins and minerals, including vitamin C.

Bean Soup

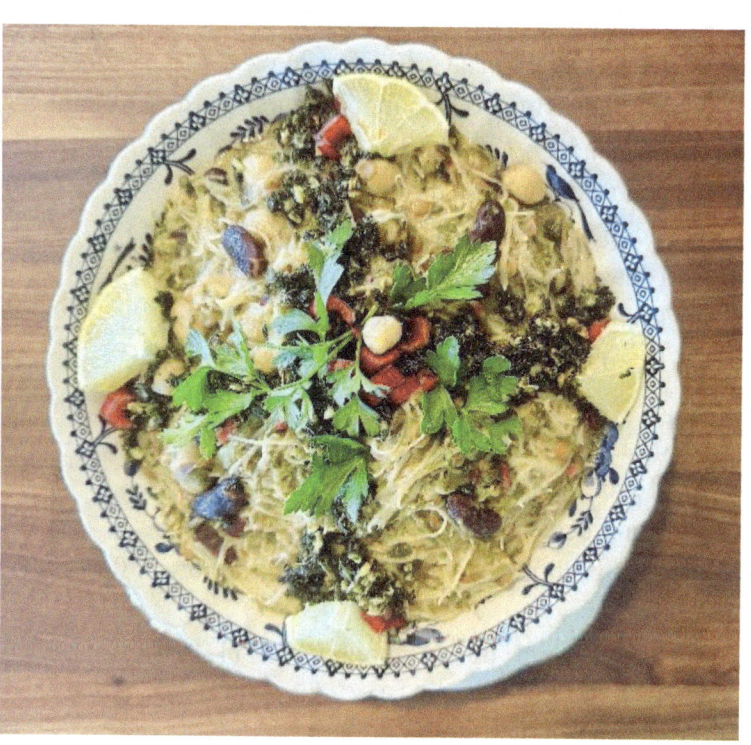

Cooking time: 40 minutes
Preparation Time: 40 minutes
Serves: 4

Ingredients:
- 1 cup lentils, 200g (7.05 oz.)
- 1 cup chickpeas, 190g (6.7 oz.)
- 1 cup kidney beans, 177g (6.24 oz.)
- 2 cups mixed chopped parsley and cilantro (coriander), 120g (4.23 oz.)
- 2 tablespoons dried mint, 30g (1 oz.)
- 1 cup homemade hummus, 480g (16.93 oz.)
- 1 teaspoon garlic powder, 5g (0.11 oz.)
- 1 teaspoon onion powder, 5g (0.11 oz.)
- 1 cup chopped onion, 150g (5.29 oz.)
- ½ teaspoon cayenne pepper (optional), 2.5g (0.04 oz.)
- ½ cup olive oil, 120g (4.23 oz.)
- 1 cup beetroot shoots, 35g (1.23 oz.)
- ¼ cup chopped parsley (for decoration), 30g (1.06 oz)
- ½ cup chives or spring onion, 40g (1.41 oz.)
- 1 cup rice noodles, 110g (3.88 oz.)
- 8 cups water, 1.89 liters (64 Fl oz.)
- 1 teaspoon dried mint (for decoration), 5g (0.04 oz.)
- 4 cloves of garlic, minced and mixed with dried mint (for decoration)
- 2-3 tablespoons lemon juice, 30-45g (1-1.5 oz.)
- Salt and pepper to taste

Recipe:

In this recipe, if you use dry beans, soak them overnight. Soaking beans can double their size, allowing enzymes to break down non-digestible sugars that cause gas in our digestive system. The best way to cook beans is to pressure-cook them. Alternatively, if you don't have much time to prepare and cook beans, use canned beans and choose brands free of BPA (bisphenol A), which can disrupt hormonal balance and is best avoided.

1. In a pan, fry the chopped onions in good-quality olive oil over a low flame until translucent.
2. Add the spices and chopped herbs to the onions.
3. In a large pot, combine the cooked beans and lentils. Add the onion and the herb mixture, then cook for 20 minutes.
4. Add *hummus (recipe indicated below) to the mix. Then add the rice noodles.
5. Allow the mixture to cook for an additional 20 minutes.
6. Adjust the water as needed to achieve the desired consistency of the soup. Add the juice of one to two whole lemons and garnish with chopped parsley, dried mint, and fried minced garlic.
7. The soup can be divided into small Pyrex containers and frozen. Thaw each portion as needed.

Everyone's tolerance for beans varies. Lectins are carbohydrate-binding proteins found in certain foods that bind to specific sugar molecules. The highest concentrations of lectins are found in healthy foods such as legumes, grains, and nightshade vegetables. Fortunately, there are several ways to reduce the lectin content of these nutritious foods to make them safer: soaking the beans in water for several hours, discarding the water, and thoroughly cooking the beans and lentils. Pressure cooking is the best way to cook beans. Sprouting and fermenting beans also reduces lectin content. Some foods, such as nightshades, contain lectins in their seeds and skin, so discarding these parts can help increase tolerance to these foods. One more tip for some individuals: beans may be easier to digest when eaten earlier in the day.

*Homemade hummus can be prepared quickly with a can of organic chickpeas, four cloves of garlic, four tablespoons of lemon juice, two tablespoons of Tahini (a sesame seed paste available in stores), a tablespoon of olive oil, additional water for a smooth consistency, salt, pepper, and any other spices you like. Mix all the ingredients in a blender and store in a glass jar in the refrigerator for up to five days. Use as a spread or add to soups and sauces.

Total Nutritional Values of Bean Soup:

Total Calories: 3700 Kcal
Total Protein: 120g
Total Carbohydrates: 300g
Total Fat: 250g
Total Dietary Fiber: 76g

Carrot And Porridge Soup

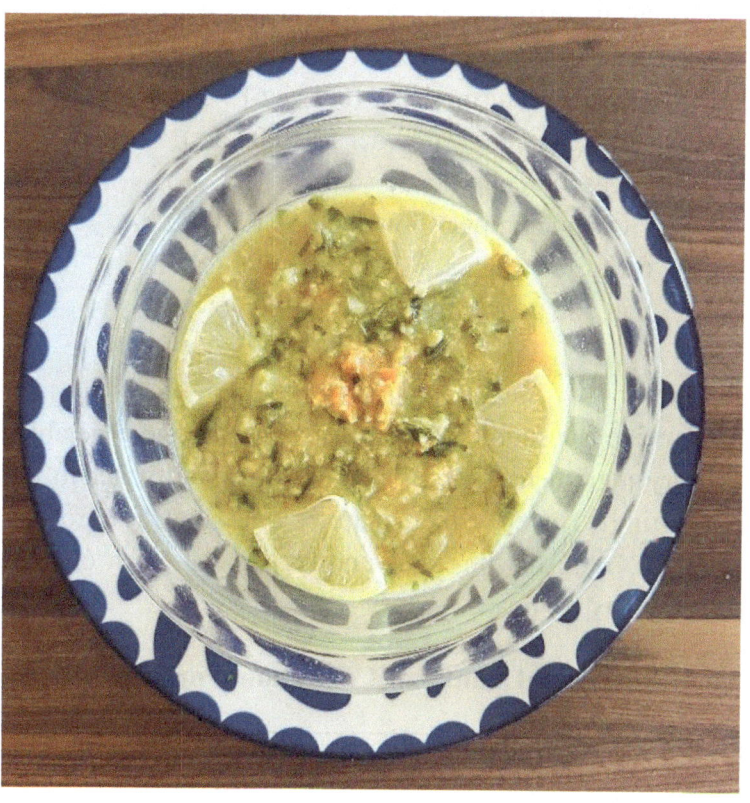

Preparation Time: 15 minutes
Cooking Time: 30 minutes
Serves: 6

Ingredients:
- ✓ 1 cup chopped organic carrots, 128g (4.5 oz.)
- ✓ 1 cup oats or porridge, 90g (3.2 oz.)
- ✓ 1 cup chopped beetroot shoots 50g (1.8 oz.)
- ✓ ½ cup organic tomato sauce (120g, 4.2 oz.)
- ✓ ½ cup chopped parsley 15g (0.5 oz.)
- ✓ 1 teaspoon turmeric 5g (0.07 oz.)
- ✓ 1 teaspoon curry powder 5g (0.07 oz.)
- ✓ 1 teaspoon paprika 5g (0.07 oz.)
- ✓ 1 teaspoon ginger powder 2.5g (0.07 oz.)
- ✓ 6 cups of water 1.4 liters (1.4 L or 48 Fl oz.)
- ✓ Salt and pepper to taste

Recipe:

This recipe is a simple one-pot dish. Chop all the vegetables and dry ingredients. Mix the spices, then add water to the pot. Bring to a boil, then simmer over low heat for 25 minutes. Garnish with herbs and serve on its own or with organic toasted bread.

Total Nutritional Values of Carrot and Porridge Soup:

Total Calories: 335 calories
Total Protein: 12g
Total Carbohydrates: 75g
Total Fat: 3g
Total Dietary Fiber: 16g

Carrots are rich in vitamins A and K and also provide vitamin C and various B vitamins. They contain minerals such as potassium, manganese, and small amounts of calcium and iron. Oats provide essential nutrients, including manganese, phosphorus, magnesium, and dietary fiber. Beetroot shoots are a rich source of vitamins A and K, as well as minerals such as potassium and calcium. Tomato sauce provides vitamins A, C, and K, as well as potassium and small amounts of iron. Parsley is rich in vitamin K and provides vitamins A and C. It also contains potassium, along with small amounts of calcium and iron. Turmeric contains curcumin, which is known for its potential health benefits.

The nutritional content of curry powder can vary based on its ingredients. It may contain small amounts of vitamins and minerals. Paprika contains multiple vitamins and minerals, including vitamins A and E. Ginger contains small amounts of vitamins, such as vitamin B6 (Pyridoxine), and minerals like potassium. Fresh lime provides vitamin C and minerals such as potassium.

The antioxidant content is primarily contributed by ingredients such as carrots (beta-carotene), parsley (vitamin C), and turmeric (curcumin), all of which are well known for their antioxidant properties. Tomatoes also provide antioxidants, including lycopene.

Tortilla Coconut Tofu Cubes

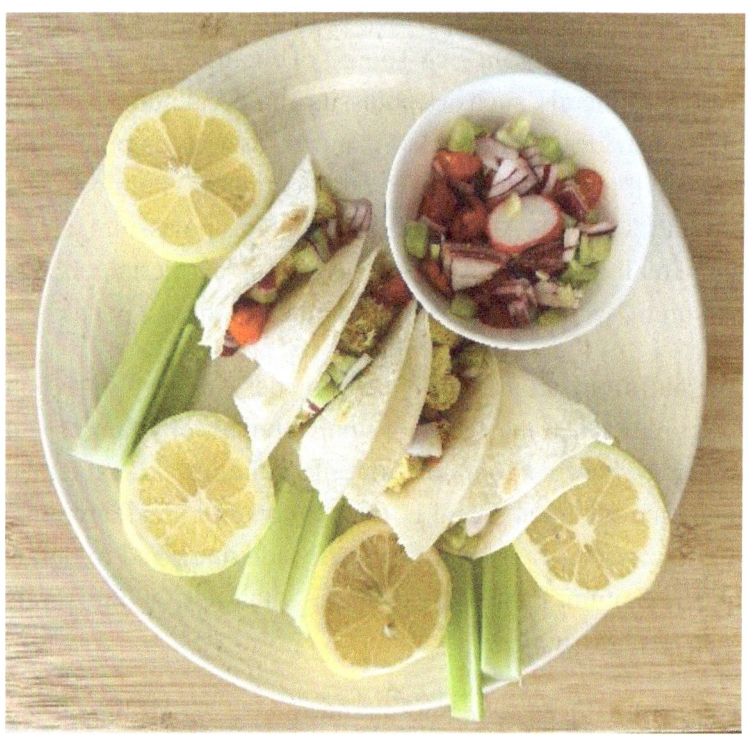

Preparation Time: 15 minutes
Cooking Time: 20 minutes
Serves: 4

Ingredients:
- ✓ 1 tub or 250g of organic tofu, cubed into small pieces
- ✓ 3 tablespoons (45 ml) of good-quality olive oil
- ✓ 1 teaspoon turmeric (5g)
- ✓ 1 teaspoon curry powder (5g)
- ✓ 1 teaspoon ginger powder (5g)
- ✓ 1 cup of organic reduced-fat unsweetened finely shredded coconut (80g or 2.8oz.)
- ✓ 2 teaspoons organic honey or maple syrup for the Vegan option (10 g or 0.35 oz.)
- ✓ 1 teaspoon garlic powder (5g)
- ✓ 2 tablespoons organic tahini (30g or 1 oz.)
- ✓ 1 pack of non-GMO or organic tortillas (typically 8-10 tortillas)
- ✓ Salt and pepper to taste

Recipe:
1. Mix all the spices and sprinkle them over the tofu cubes.
2. Add the olive oil and honey (maple syrup for the Vegan option) to the surface of the tofu.
3. Gently place the shredded dried coconut on a plate, then roll the tofu cubes in the coconut to coat them with coconut and spices.
4. Place parchment paper on the oven tray, then arrange the tofu cubes.
5. Bake at 350 degrees for 10 minutes.

6. The tofu cubes can be served on toasted tortillas, drizzled with honey or tahini, or with maple syrup for the vegan option, alongside a salad of tomatoes, onions, cucumbers, and mixed organic greens.

Total Nutritional Values of Tortilla Coconut Tofu Cubes

Total Calories: 1,106 Kcal
Total Protein: 30g
Total Carbohydrates: 40g
Total Fat: 98g
Total Dietary Fiber: 12g

Tofu is a good source of protein and provides essential minerals, including calcium, iron, and magnesium. It also contains small amounts of vitamins, such as vitamin K.

Olive oil is a good source of monounsaturated fats, vitamins E and K, and other nutrients discussed earlier. Turmeric contains curcumin, which is known for its potential health benefits. Ginger contains small amounts of vitamins, such as vitamin B6 (Pyridoxine), and minerals, including potassium. Coconut contains small amounts of vitamins, such as folate. It also contains minerals such as manganese, small amounts of iron, and copper.

Honey contains 45 kcal per tablespoon and 10-12 g of carbohydrates. The health benefits of honey are largely attributed to its antioxidant content and its physical properties.

Raw and darker varieties of honey contain antioxidants, including flavonoids and phenolic acids. These compounds help neutralize unstable molecules (free radicals) in the body, which can contribute to overall health and protection against cell damage.

For the Vegan option, use maple syrup. Tahini provides minerals such as calcium and iron, as well as small amounts of B vitamins. One pack of non-GMO tortillas: calorie and nutritional values may vary by type and brand.

Mushroom and Tofu Stew

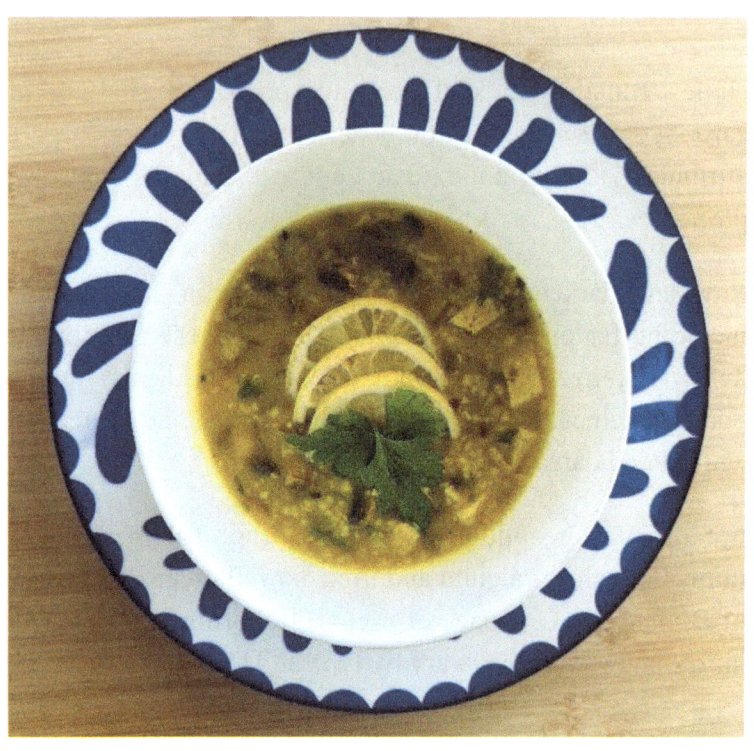

Preparation Time: 15-20 minutes (including chopping and soaking)
Cooking Time: 30-40 minutes
Serves: 4

Ingredients:
- ✓ 1 cup of Portobello mushrooms, or any other mushroom available, chopped (100g or 3.5oz.)
- ✓ ½ cup chopped parsley (15g or 0.5 oz.)
- ✓ ½ cup of steel-cut oats, soaked overnight (90g or 3.2oz.)
- ✓ ½ teaspoon turmeric (2.5g)
- ✓ ½ teaspoon curry powder (2.5g)
- ✓ ½ cup chopped organic tofu (125g or 4.4oz.)
- ✓ 1 medium-sized onion, chopped (150g or 5.3oz.)
- ✓ 1 tablespoon olive oil (15 ml)
- ✓ 4-5 cups of water (950-1200 ml)
- ✓ One whole Lemon juice
- ✓ Salt and pepper to taste

Recipe:
1. Pour one tablespoon of good-quality olive oil into a pan, then add the chopped onions.
2. Fry the onions until golden, then add the mushrooms, tofu cubes, parsley, and spices.
3. Let the mushrooms and tofu simmer for 5 minutes.
4. In a medium pot, combine the oats and water. Bring the mixture to a boil, then reduce the heat and simmer for 15 minutes.
5. Add the tofu, mushrooms, and herbs to the pot, then season with salt and pepper as needed.
6. Add lemon juice before serving.
7. The stew can be served on its own or with salad and organic toasted bread.

Total Nutritional Values of Mushroom and Tofu Stew

Total Calories: 448 calories Total Protein: 19g Total Carbohydrates: 48g Total Fat: 23g Total Dietary Fiber: 9g

Portobello mushrooms are a good source of vitamin D and Riboflavin (B2) and provide small amounts of other B vitamins. They contain essential minerals such as potassium, phosphorus, copper, and selenium. Parsley is rich in vitamin K and provides vitamins A and C. It contains minerals such as potassium, along with small amounts of calcium and iron. Oats provide nutrients like manganese, phosphorus, and magnesium. Turmeric contains curcumin, which is known for its potential health benefits. Curry powder contains small amounts of various vitamins and minerals. Tofu provides small amounts of vitamins like vitamin K and Riboflavin (B2). It contains essential minerals, including calcium, iron, and magnesium. Onions offer vitamins C and B6 (Pyridoxine), minerals such as potassium, and small amounts of manganese and copper. Olive oil provides mainly healthy monounsaturated fats and vitamins E and K.

Garlic Avocado Pesto

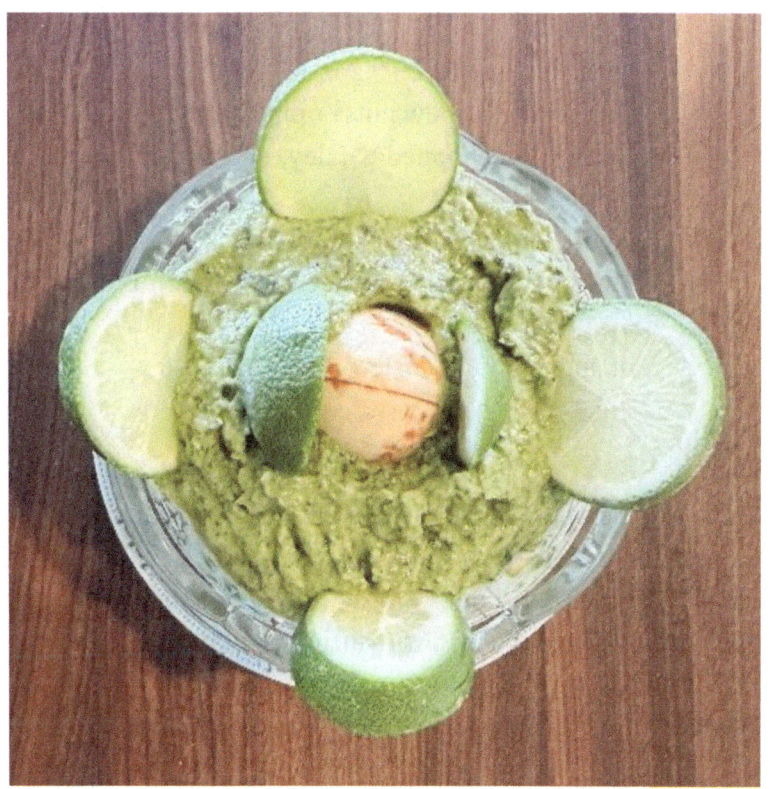

Preparation Time: 10-15 minutes (including peeling avocados and juicing lemons)
Cooking Time: None
Serves: 4

Ingredients:

- ✓ 4-5 whole avocados, peeled, and pitted (400g or 14oz.)
- ✓ 2 garlic cloves (6g or 0.2oz.)
- ✓ ½ cup of raw cashew nuts or pine nuts (70g or 2.5oz.)
- ✓ 1 tablespoon chopped parsley, cilantro, or coriander (15g or ½ oz.)
- ✓ 2 whole lemons, juiced (60ml or two Fl oz.)
- ✓ 1 tablespoon good quality olive oil (15ml or 0.5 Fl oz.)
- ✓ Salt and pepper to taste

Recipe:

Mix all the ingredients in a blender, then transfer to a container suitable for refrigeration. This spread can be used as an alternative to butter on sandwiches. It can be kept in the fridge for a few days in an airtight container.

Total Nutritional Values of Garlic Avocado Pesto

Total Calories: 1,050 Kcal
Total Protein: 20g
Total Carbohydrates: 65g
Total Fat: 89g
Total Dietary Fiber: 27g

Avocados contain multiple polyphenols, including flavonoids such as quercetin and kaempferol. They are rich in potassium, vitamin K, and vitamin E. They also provide small amounts of vitamins C, B6 (pyridoxine), and B9 (folate), as well as minerals such as potassium, magnesium, and copper, and are a good source of fiber. Garlic contains small amounts of vitamins C and B9 (folate). It also contains minerals like manganese, along with small amounts of calcium and iron. Raw cashew nuts or pine nuts are rich in vitamin E and magnesium and provide small amounts of B vitamins. Parsley and cilantro are rich in vitamin K and provide vitamins A and C. They also contain minerals like potassium, along with small amounts of calcium and iron. Lemons are a good source of vitamin C, provide small amounts of vitamins B6 (pyridoxine) and B9 (folate), and contain minerals like potassium. Good-quality olive oil contains mainly healthy monounsaturated fats, vitamins E and K, and polyphenols.

Mushroom Omelet

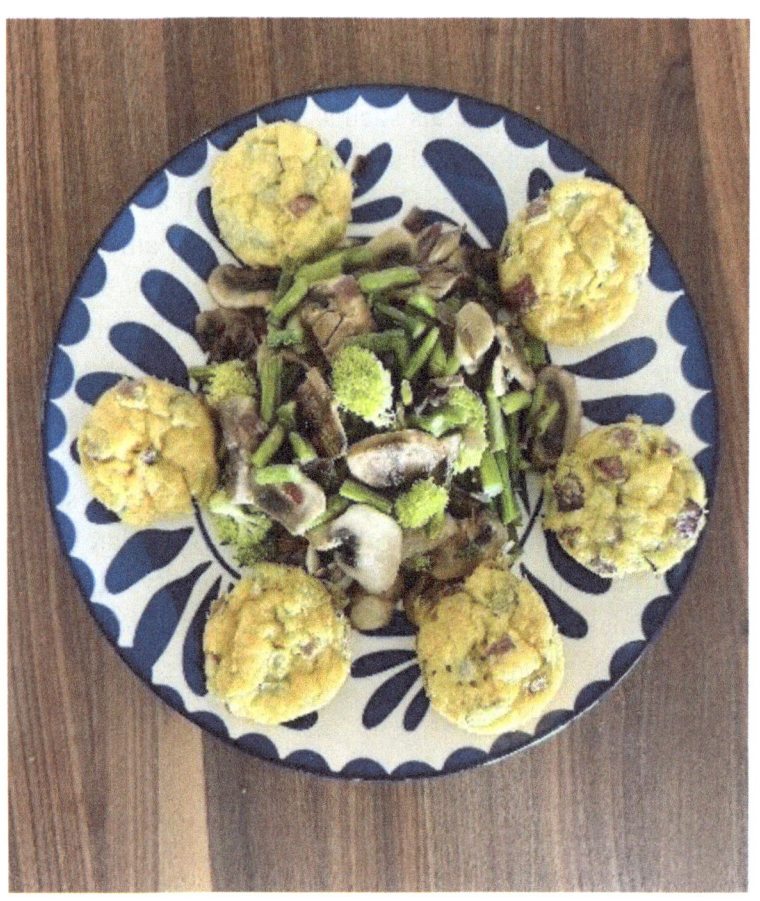

Preparation Time: 15-20 minutes (including chopping vegetables and herbs)
Cooking Time: 25 minutes
Serves: 2

Ingredients:
- ✓ ½ cup (50g or 1.8oz.) chopped portobello mushrooms (or any other kind)
- ✓ 2 organic pasture-raised eggs
- ✓ ½ cup (60g or 2.1oz.) chopped asparagus
- ✓ ½ cup (60g or 2.1oz.) chopped broccoli
- ✓ ½ cup (30g or 1 oz) chopped mixed herbs (parsley and basil)
- ✓ 1 teaspoon turmeric (2g)
- ✓ 1 tablespoon rice flour (15g or ½oz.)
- ✓ ½ teaspoon baking powder (2.5g)
- ✓ ½ cup (75g or 2.6oz.) chopped onion
- ✓ 2 tablespoons (30ml) good-quality olive oil
- ✓ Salt and pepper to taste

Recipe:
1. In a medium-sized pan, add a generous amount of high-quality olive oil.
2. Add the chopped onions to the pan and cook them until they are golden.
3. Next, add the chopped mushrooms to the pan and let them brown over medium heat for 10 minutes, along with the chopped asparagus and broccoli.
4. Mix the organic eggs with the mixed herbs and spices, baking powder, and flour in a large bowl until well combined.
5. In a muffin baking pan, pour the egg mixture into each segment.

6. Place it in the oven and bake at 350°F for 15 minutes. Add salt and pepper to taste. Serve it on its own for breakfast or a simple lunch.

Vegan Option
1. In a medium-sized pan, add a generous amount of good-quality olive oil.
2. Add the chopped onions and let them turn golden.
3. Then, add the spices and chopped mushrooms, allowing them to turn golden, along with the chopped asparagus and broccoli.
4. Add ½ a tub of tofu, cut into cubes, to the vegetable mixture. Cook the mixture over a medium flame for 10 minutes.
5. It can be served with a salad or used to make a sandwich with organic bread.

Total Nutritional Values of mushroom Omelet	Vegan Nutritional Value
Total Calories: 447 Kcal Total Protein: 17g Total Carbohydrates: 16g Total Fat: 38g Total Dietary Fiber: 3g	Total Calories: 539 Kcal Total Protein: 24.7g Total Carbohydrates: 36g Total Fat: 36.2g Total Fiber: 8.8g

Portabella mushrooms are a good source of vitamin D and riboflavin (B2) and provide small amounts of other B vitamins. They also contain minerals such as potassium and phosphorus, along with small amounts of copper and selenium. Eggs are a good source of vitamin B12 and provide vitamins A and D. They contain minerals like selenium and small amounts of iron. Asparagus is rich in vitamin K and provides vitamins A, C, and folate. It also contains minerals like potassium and small amounts of iron. Broccoli is a good source of vitamin C and provides vitamins A and K. It contains minerals such as potassium, as well as small amounts of calcium and iron. Chopped herbs, such as parsley and basil, provide negligible calories and carbohydrates. Herbs like parsley and basil are rich in vitamins A and K and provide small amounts of vitamin C. They contain minerals such as potassium, along with small amounts of calcium and iron. Turmeric contains curcumin, which is known for its potential health benefits. Onions contain vitamins C and B6 (Pyridoxine). Onions also provide minerals like potassium, small amounts of manganese and copper, and quercetin. Good-quality olive oil is mainly made up of healthy monounsaturated fats. It also contains vitamins E and K. The antioxidant content of this recipe comes from ingredients such as turmeric, asparagus, broccoli, parsley, and basil, all recognized for their antioxidant properties.

Lemony Shiitake Stew

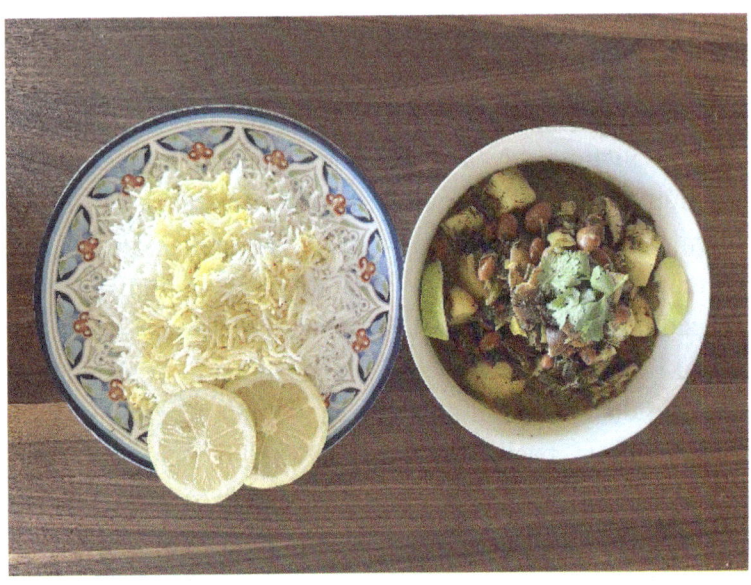

Preparation Time: 30-40 minutes (including chopping vegetables and herbs)
Cooking Time: 30-40 minutes
Serves: 4

Ingredients:
- ✓ 1 cup (70 grams or 2.5 ounces) of sliced shiitake mushrooms or any other mushrooms available
- ✓ 1 medium-sized onion (150 grams or 5.3 ounces), chopped
- ✓ 1 cup (100 grams or 3.5 ounces) green onions, finely chopped
- ✓ 2 cups (60 grams or 2.1 ounces) parsley, finely chopped
- ✓ 1 cup (30 grams or 1 ounce) cilantro (coriander), finely chopped
- ✓ 1 cup (30 grams or 1 ounce) chopped leek or spring onion
- ✓ 1 tablespoon dried fenugreek (usually available in international stores)
- ✓ 1 cup (200 grams or 7 ounces) cooked organic pinto beans
- ✓ 2 medium organic potatoes (400 grams or 14 ounces), cut into similar-sized segments
- ✓ 8 tablespoons (120 ml or four fluid ounces) good-quality olive oil
- ✓ ½ cup (120 ml or four fluid ounces) fresh lime juice
- ✓ 2 or 3 dried limes, crushed (optional, usually available in international stores)
- ✓ 1 tablespoon non-GMO corn flour (cornstarch) (15 grams or ½ ounce)
- ✓ 1 teaspoon curry powder (2 grams)
- ✓ 1 teaspoon turmeric (5 grams)

- ✓ 1 teaspoon paprika (5 grams)
- ✓ 2 fresh lemons, juiced (60 ml or two fluid ounces)
- ✓ Salt and pepper to taste
- ✓ Pinch of saffron, crushed and mixed with one tablespoon of water

Recipe:
1. Wash the mushrooms and slice them.
2. In a large pan, pour two tablespoons of good-quality olive oil.
3. Add the chopped onion and leeks and cook until they become translucent.
4. Add the chopped herbs and spices to the large pan, along with the onions and leeks, then add four tablespoons of olive oil. Cook over low heat for 35 minutes, or until the mixture reduces in volume.
5. Add two tablespoons of good-quality olive oil to a separate pan and fry the chopped potatoes over a low flame for 10 to 15 minutes, or until cooked through.
6. Add the mushroom slices to the pan.
7. Transfer the mushroom and potato mixture to the large pan along with all the herbal blends.
8. Add some water with corn flour to the mix in the large pan.
9. Add the cooked organic beans and some dried lime if available; alternatively, fresh lemon can be used.
10. Add a pinch of saffron and cook the mixture for 20 minutes. This dish has a fantastic aroma of herbs and spices that fills the air.

11. Add lemon, salt, and pepper as required.

I am creating a vegetarian version of this dish, which was originally made with lamb. It can be served over steamed basmati rice with a salad.

Total Nutritional Values of Lemony Shiitake Stew

Total Calories: 1609 Kcal
Total Protein: 32g
Total Carbohydrates: 146g
Total Fat: 115g
Total Dietary Fiber: 47g

Shiitake mushrooms provide vitamins such as vitamin D, B vitamins, and small amounts of vitamin C. They contain minerals such as selenium and copper, along with small amounts of iron and zinc. Onions contain vitamins C and B6 (Pyridoxine). Onions also provide minerals such as potassium, as well as small amounts of manganese and copper. Spring onions and leeks offer vitamins A and K, as well as minerals such as potassium, and contain small amounts of calcium and iron. Parsley is rich in vitamin K and provides vitamins A and C. It contains minerals such as potassium, calcium, and iron. Cilantro delivers vitamins A and K. It contains minerals such as potassium, as well as small amounts of calcium and iron. Beans are a rich source of various vitamins and minerals, including folate, potassium, and iron. Potatoes are a source of vitamin C and provide small amounts of vitamins B6 (Pyridoxine) and B9 (Folate). They contain minerals such as potassium, along with small amounts of magnesium and iron. Olive oil (mainly healthy monounsaturated fats) also provides vitamin E.

Lime juice provides vitamin C and essential minerals, including potassium. Curry powder can vary in composition based on the ingredients and may contain small amounts of vitamins and minerals. Turmeric contains curcumin, which is known for its potential health benefits. Paprika contains several vitamins and minerals, including vitamins A and E. A pinch of saffron provides negligible calories and carbohydrates and has antioxidant properties.

Various ingredients, including shiitake mushrooms, parsley, coriander, and spices such as turmeric, paprika, and saffron, contribute to the recipe's antioxidant content.

Heavenly Saffron Steamed Basmati Rice

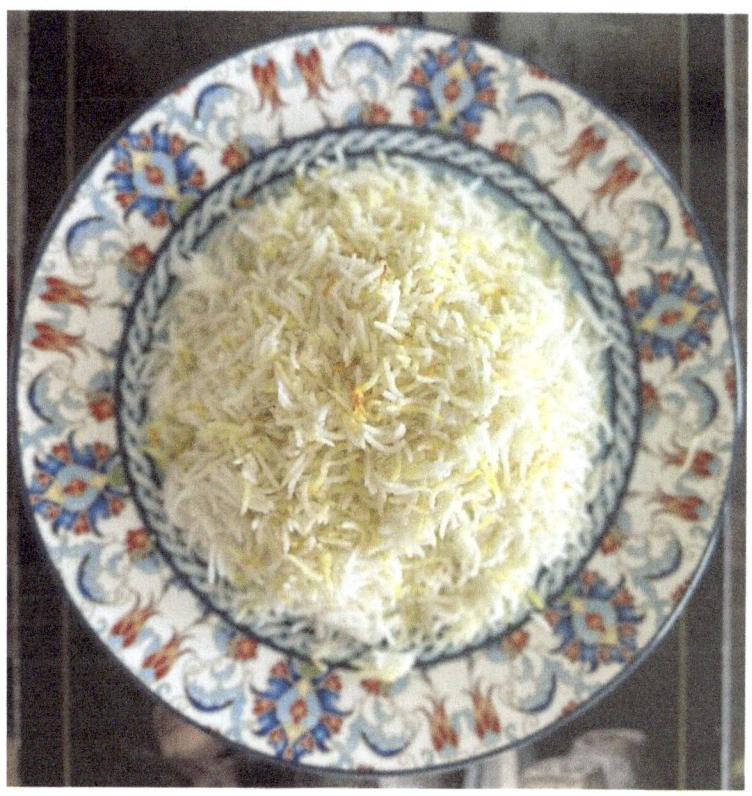

Preparation Time: 5-10 minutes, washing rice and preparing saffron if available
Cooking Time: 20-30 minutes for boiling rice
Serves: 4-6

Ingredients:
- ✓ 2 cups Basmati rice, washed (400 g / 14 oz.)
- ✓ 8–10 cups water (1.9–2.4 L) for boiling
- ✓ 2 tablespoons of olive oil (30 ml / 1 Fl oz)
- ✓ 1 teaspoon of saffron, crushed (0.5 g)
- ✓ Salt to taste

Recipe:
1. Wash the basmati rice under cold water, then soak the grains in a bowl of cold water for at least an hour. If time is limited, you can proceed with the recipe immediately after washing the rice a few times.
2. Boil 2 liters (about 8 to 10 cups) of water in a pan, then add the rice. At this stage, it will take only 5-10 minutes for the rice grains to double in size. To test readiness, take a rice grain and break it in half with your finger. It should break easily, not too quickly or too hard.
3. Remove the pan from the stove, drain the rice in a colander, and sprinkle with salt.
4. Put the pan back on the stove, add two tablespoons of good-quality olive oil, reduce the heat to low, and return the parboiled rice to the pan.
5. Let it steam for at least 20 minutes. Traditionally, a clean cloth is wrapped securely around the pan lid to prevent further condensation.
6. Place the saffron strands in a mortar and crush them into a fine powder. Add a tablespoon of water. Mix well.

7. When the rice is ready to serve, pour the mortar's contents over the rice.
8. The rice at the bottom of the pan turns crispy after 20 minutes over a medium-low flame and tastes very good!
9. One can serve this rice on a platter.

Basmati rice can accompany some of the dishes listed in the book. White rice can be replaced with brown or wild rice, but keep in mind that it will take longer to cook. Brown and wild rice take longer to boil, and the water-to-rice ratio is higher. Soak the rice grains overnight; alternatively, consider a mixture of half white rice and half brown rice. Brown rice requires more cooking time. Adding salt to the rice after boiling is a better way to preserve the B vitamins, which are unstable in alkaline solutions.

Cooking rice in a rice cooker is easier and saves time. In that case, one must follow the rice cooker's instructions for the water-to-rice ratio.

Total Nutritional Values for Steamed Basmati Rice Recipe

Total Calories: 1600 Kcal
Total Protein: 30 g
Total Carbohydrates: 312 g
Total Fat: 32 g
Total Dietary Fiber: 8 g

Basmati rice is a good source of carbohydrates and provides small amounts of vitamins and minerals, such as thiamine (B1) and niacin (B3). It also contains minerals such as magnesium and phosphorus.

Olive oil contains mainly healthy monounsaturated fats and vitamins E and K.

One teaspoon of **Saffron** (crushed) provides negligible calories and carbohydrates. Saffron is primarily used for its flavor and color. Saffron contains many antioxidant compounds, such as Crocin and Crocetin. Just a few strands bring about extra nutritional value to the dish you are cooking.

Embrace The Young You

Nutty Split Pea Stew

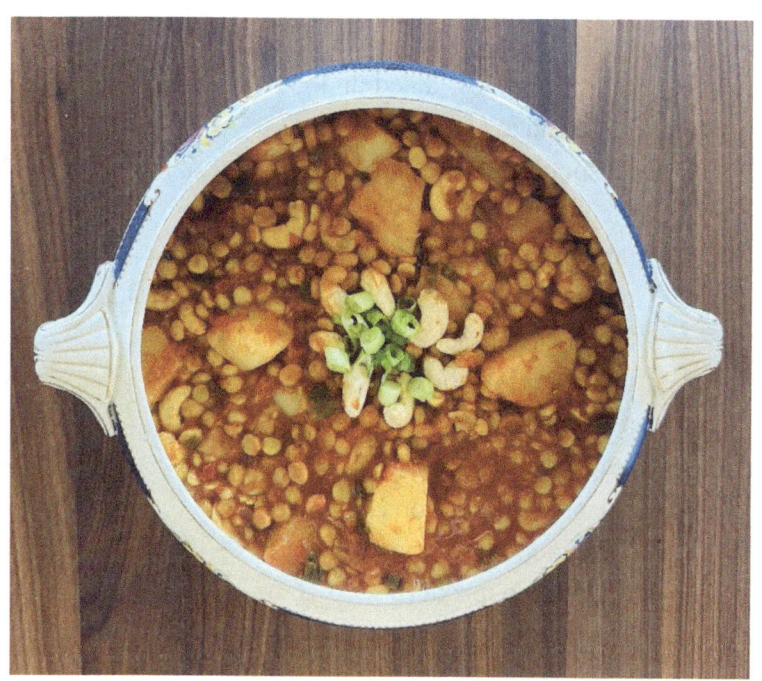

Total Preparation Time: 25-30 minutes
Total Cooking Time: 30-40 minutes
Serves: 4-6

Ingredients:
- ✓ 1 cup split peas (200 g / 7 oz.)
- ✓ 1/2 lb. tomatoes, diced and grated, or 1 cup organic tomato sauce (400 g / 14 oz.)
- ✓ 2 teaspoons tomato puree (10 g / 0.7 oz.)
- ✓ 2 medium-sized potatoes, diced (300 g / 11.5 oz.)
- ✓ 4 tablespoons olive oil (60 g / 2 oz.)
- ✓ 1 medium-sized red onion, diced (150 g / 5.3 oz.)
- ✓ 1/2 cup cashew nuts (75 g / 2.6 oz.)
- ✓ 1 teaspoon nutritional yeast (5 g / 0.1 oz.)
- ✓ 1 teaspoon curry powder (5 g / 0.16 oz.)
- ✓ 1 teaspoon turmeric (5 g / 0.16 oz.)
- ✓ 1 teaspoon cinnamon (5 g / 0.16 oz.)
- ✓ 1/2 teaspoon cayenne pepper (2.5 g / 0.08 oz.)
- ✓ 1 teaspoon paprika (5 g / 0.16 oz.)
- ✓ Salt and pepper to taste

Recipe:
1. Soak the split peas for at least an hour beforehand.
2. Cook the split peas in a saucepan for 30 minutes, or until tender. Make sure the split peas are not overcooked.
3. Drain the peas and set them aside. *If dried lime is available, pour boiling water over it and let it sit for 30 minutes. If dried lime is unavailable, fresh lemon juice can be used as an alternative.*
4. In a saucepan, heat olive oil and add diced onions, letting them turn golden.

5. Add the spices, tomato puree, and tomato sauce. Then add the juice from the dried lime (optional), and pour one cup of water into the pot.
6. Let the mixture cook for 20 minutes, then add the cooked split peas and cook for an additional 10 minutes over low heat.
7. While the stew is cooking, place the diced potatoes in a frying pan and cook them in olive oil over a low flame for 10 minutes, or until cooked through.
8. Add the diced potatoes to the split-pea and tomato mixture in the saucepan, then boil for 10 minutes.
9. Add the cashews and nutritional yeast, then sprinkle with chopped parsley for decoration.
10. Add salt and pepper to taste.

The dish can be served on its own or over basmati rice for a more substantial meal, accompanied by a mixed salad.

Total Nutritional Values for Nutty Split Pea Stew

Total Calories: 2050 Kcal
Total Protein: 75g
Total Carbohydrates: 195g
Total Fat: 120 g
Total Dietary Fiber: 45g

Split peas provide vitamins B1 (thiamine), B5 (pantothenic acid), and B9 (folate). They contain essential minerals such as potassium, magnesium, and iron. Tomatoes are a good source of vitamin C and provide small amounts of vitamin A, vitamin K, and folate. They contain minerals such as potassium, along with small amounts of manganese and copper. Tomato puree provides vitamins such as C and small amounts of K and folate. It contains minerals such as potassium, along with small amounts of manganese and copper. Potatoes are a good source of vitamin C and provide vitamins B6 (pyridoxine) and B9 (folate). They contain minerals such as potassium, along with small amounts of magnesium and iron. Onions contain vitamins C and B6 (pyridoxine). They also provide minerals such as potassium, along with small amounts of manganese and copper. Cashew nuts are a rich source of vitamins, including vitamin K and E, and provide essential minerals such as magnesium and copper. Nutritional yeast is fortified with B vitamins, including B12, and contains minerals such as zinc. Turmeric contains curcumin, which is known for its potential health benefits.

Cinnamon contains small amounts of vitamins and minerals, including vitamin K and calcium. Cayenne pepper is a source of vitamin A and provides small amounts of vitamin C. Paprika contains vitamins A and E. Olive oil (mainly monounsaturated fats) contains vitamins E and K.

Lime juice provides vitamin C and essential minerals, including potassium. This recipe has anti-inflammatory and antioxidant properties, thanks to the combination of beans, nuts, and spices. The dish also contains soluble fiber from the split peas. The tomato-based dish contains the antioxidant lycopene, which has been shown to have an anti-aging effect. The lime's acidity helps preserve the potato's vitamin C and improve iron absorption. Cashew nuts and split peas are good sources of protein and minerals.

Tomatoes contain the antioxidant lycopene and vitamin C. The dish's acidity aids iron absorption. Capsaicin, the compound that gives cayenne peppers their pungency, also enhances curcumin absorption from turmeric. Research shows that capsaicin boosts the body's ability to break down fat and burn more energy. This dish is high in fiber.

Spicy Red Lentil Stew

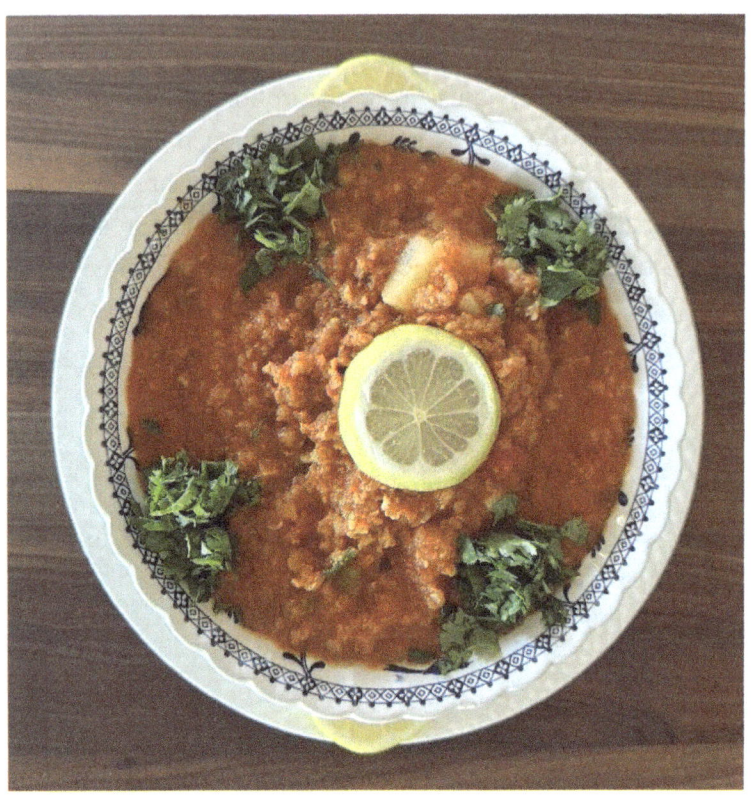

Total Preparation time: 25-30 minutes
Total Cooking time: 25-30 minutes
Serves: 4-6

Ingredients:
- ✓ 1/2 lb. or 1 cup red lentils (225 g / 8 oz.)
- ✓ 4 cloves garlic, minced (12 g / 0.4 oz.)
- ✓ 4 medium-sized tomatoes (600 g / 21 oz.)
- ✓ 1 can organic tomatoes (400 g / 14 oz) or 1 cup organic tomato sauce
- ✓ 1 medium organic potato, cut into small pieces (200 g / 7 oz.)
- ✓ 1 medium sweet potato, cut into small pieces (300 g / 10.5 oz.)
- ✓ 1 chili pepper (optional)
- ✓ 1 teaspoon of curry powder (5 g / 0.16 oz.)
- ✓ 1 teaspoon turmeric (5 g / 0.16 oz.)
- ✓ 2 tablespoons mixture of tamarind paste and tomato paste (30 g / 1 oz.)
- ✓ 2 tablespoons olive oil (30 g / 1 oz.)
- ✓ Juice of 1 lemon (30 g / 1 oz.)
- ✓ Salt and pepper to taste

Recipe:
1. Combine the lentils with water in a saucepan, then add a cup of organic tomato sauce, diced organic potatoes, and two tablespoons of tomato paste. *If tamarind is available, add a tablespoon; if not, use the tomato paste.*
2. Let it cook for 20 minutes over a medium flame.
3. In a stainless-steel frying pan, heat good-quality olive oil and add the chopped onion.

4. Once golden, add the minced garlic, green chili, and spices.
5. Grate the tomatoes into a dish, discard the seeds and skin, and add the grated tomatoes to the spice mixture.
6. Pour the mixture into the saucepan with the remaining ingredients.
7. Add salt, pepper, and lemon juice to taste, then cook for 10 minutes.

This dish can be served on its own or accompanied by a bed of basmati rice, homemade bread, and a green salad. Garnish with chopped parsley and cilantro, or coriander.

Total Nutritional Values for Spicy Red Lentil Stew

Total Calories: 2150 Kcal
Total Protein: 75g
Total Carbohydrates: 255g
Total Fat: 125g
Total Dietary Fiber: 70g

Red lentils provide vitamins such as folate, vitamin B1 (Thiamine), and vitamin B6 (Pyridoxine). They contain essential minerals such as iron, potassium, and magnesium. Garlic contains small amounts of vitamins, such as C and B6 (Pyridoxine). It provides minerals like manganese. Tomatoes are a good source of vitamin C and provide small amounts of vitamin A, vitamin K, and folate. They contain minerals such as potassium, along with small amounts of manganese and copper. Tomato sauce provides vitamins like vitamin C and small amounts of vitamin K and folate. It contains minerals such as potassium, along with small amounts of manganese and copper. Potatoes are a good source of vitamin C and provide vitamins B6 (Pyridoxine) and B9 (Folate). They contain small amounts of minerals such as magnesium and iron. Sweet potatoes are rich in vitamins A and C and provide small amounts of vitamin B5 (pantothenic acid) and B6 (Pyridoxine). They contain minerals like potassium and manganese. Chili peppers are a source of vitamins such as C and B6 (Pyridoxine). They contain minerals like potassium and small amounts of manganese. Turmeric contains curcumin, which is known for its potential health benefits. Tamarind contains vitamins such as vitamin C and small amounts of thiamine (vitamin B1). It contains minerals like potassium and magnesium. Lentils contain soluble fiber that helps stabilize blood sugar levels. Tomatoes have antioxidants and vitamin C. The dish's acidity helps with iron absorption. Spices have many anti-inflammatory effects. It is high in fiber, and pairing Basmati rice and salad with this dish can still keep the glycemic load low due to the lentils' high fiber content.

Chili Veggie Style

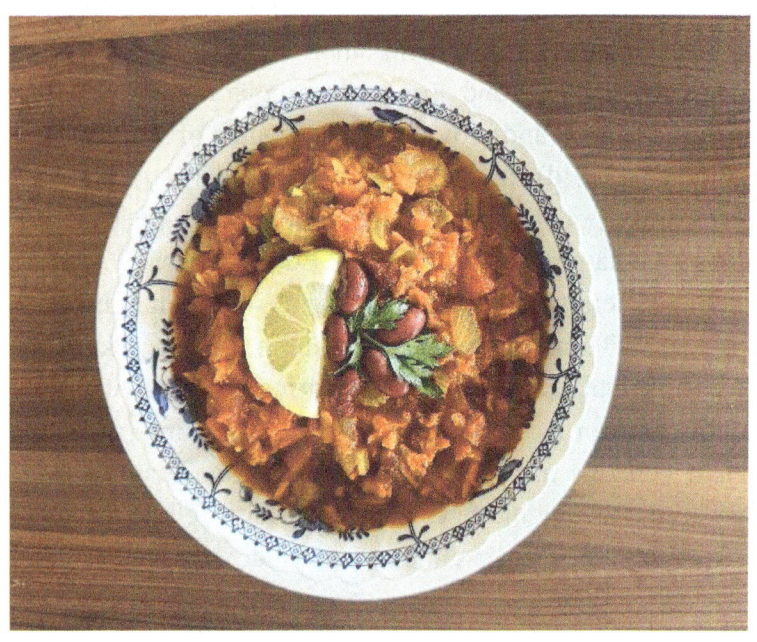

Total Preparation Time: 25-30 minutes
Total cooking time: 20-25 minutes
Serves: 4-6

Ingredients:
- ✓ ½ can organic kidney beans, cooked (125 g / 4.4 oz.)
- ✓ 1 medium-sized onion, chopped (150 g / 5.3 oz.)
- ✓ 2 carrots, shredded (200 g / 7 oz.)
- ✓ 2 stalks of organic celery, chopped (100 g / 3.5 oz.)
- ✓ 2 cloves of garlic, chopped (10 g / 0.4 oz.)
- ✓ 3 tomatoes, chopped (450 g / 16 oz.)
- ✓ 1 teaspoon chili powder (5 g / 0.16 oz.)
- ✓ 1 green chili (optional)
- ✓ 1 teaspoon turmeric (5 g / 0.16 oz.)
- ✓ 1 teaspoon curry powder (5 g / 0.16 oz.)
- ✓ 2 tablespoons tomato paste (30 g / 1 oz.)
- ✓ 1 can of organic tomatoes (250 g / 8.8 oz.)
- ✓ Juice of 1 fresh lemon (30 g / 1 oz.)
- ✓ 2 tablespoons extra virgin olive oil (30 g / 1 oz.)
- ✓ Salt and pepper to taste

Recipe:
1. Fry the diced onion in good-quality olive oil. Once it turns golden, add the chopped garlic, shredded carrots, celery, and all the spices.
2. Add tomato paste, one can of organic tomatoes, and cooked organic beans, then let the mixture simmer for 15 minutes.
3. Add salt and pepper to taste and lemon juice as needed. The dish can be served over basmati rice or on its own.
4. Store in small Pyrex dishes in the freezer.

Total Nutritional Values for Chili Veggie Style

Total Calories: 750 Kcal
Total Protein: 30g
Total Carbohydrates: 140g
Total Fat: 32g
Total Dietary Fiber: 38g

Kidney beans provide vitamins such as folate and small amounts of vitamins B1 (Thiamine) and B6 (Pyridoxine). They contain essential minerals such as potassium, magnesium, and iron. Onions contain vitamins C and B6 (Pyridoxine) and provide minerals such as potassium, along with small amounts of manganese and copper. Carrots are a good source of vitamin A and provide vitamins K and C. They contain minerals such as potassium and small amounts of manganese. Celery offers vitamins A and K. It contains potassium and small amounts of calcium and magnesium. Garlic contains small amounts of vitamin B6 (Pyridoxine). It provides minerals such as manganese, along with small amounts of calcium and iron.

Tomatoes are a good source of vitamin C and provide small amounts of vitamin A, vitamin K, and folate. They contain minerals such as potassium, along with small amounts of manganese and copper. Chili powder can vary in nutritional content, but it typically includes vitamins such as vitamin A and minerals like potassium. Green chilies provide vitamin C and small amounts of vitamin B6 (Pyridoxine). They also contain minerals such as potassium. Turmeric contains curcumin, which is known for its potential health benefits. Tomato paste provides vitamins such as C and small amounts of K and folate. It contains minerals such as potassium, along with small amounts of manganese and copper. Canned tomatoes provide vitamins such as C and small amounts of K and folate. They contain minerals such as potassium, along with small amounts of manganese and copper. Lemon juice provides vitamin C and contains minerals such as potassium. Olive oil (mainly monounsaturated fats) includes vitamins E and K. This recipe offers antioxidant and anti-inflammatory benefits thanks to the powerful ingredients, including beans, spices, and vegetables. This dish is low in saturated fat and high in fiber. Beans have soluble fiber that helps stabilize blood sugar levels.

Asparagus Soup

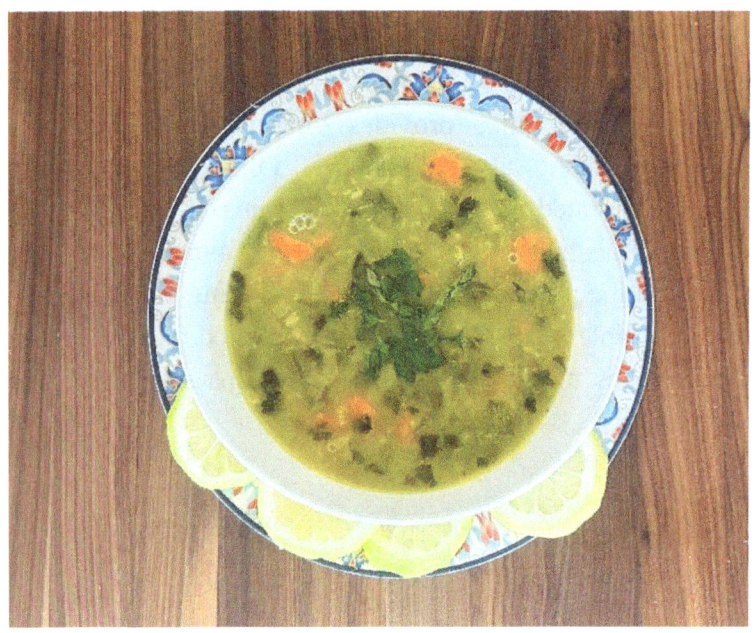

Total Preparation Time: 25-30 minutes
Total Cooking Time: 20-25 minutes
Serves: 4

Ingredients:
- ✓ 1 cup chopped fresh asparagus (150 g / 5.3 oz.)
- ✓ 1 medium-sized onion (150 g / 5.3 oz.)
- ✓ 2 medium-sized organic carrots (200 g / 7 oz.)
- ✓ 1 medium-sized organic sweet potato (200 g / 7 oz.)
- ✓ ½ cup chopped spring onions (50 g / 1.8 oz.)
- ✓ 2 tablespoons oats (20 g / 0.7 oz.)
- ✓ 1 teaspoon turmeric (3–5 g / 0.1 oz.)
- ✓ Juice of 1 fresh lime or lemon (30 g / 1 oz.)
- ✓ 2 cups of water (300 ml / 300 g / 10.6 oz.)
- ✓ 2 tablespoons chopped parsley (10 g / 0.4 oz.)
- ✓ Salt and pepper to taste

Recipe:
1. Add oats, spices, and water to the pan, bring to a boil, then reduce the heat.
2. Wash all the vegetables, chop them into small pieces, and add them to the pan with the oats and spices.
3. Allow to cook for 20 minutes.
4. Decorate with chopped herbs.

Total Nutritional Values for Asparagus Soup

Total Calories: 453 calories
Total Protein: 14g
Total Carbohydrates: 88g
Total Fat: 3g
Total Dietary Fiber: 20g

Asparagus is a good source of vitamins K and A, and also contains small amounts of vitamin C and vitamin B9 (folate). It contains minerals like potassium and small amounts of manganese. Onions contain vitamins C and B6 (pyridoxine), as well as minerals such as potassium, along with small amounts of manganese and copper. Carrots are a good source of vitamin A and provide vitamins K and C. They also contain minerals such as potassium and small amounts of manganese. Sweet potatoes are rich in vitamins A and C and provide small amounts of vitamins B5 (pantothenic acid) and B6 (pyridoxine). They contain minerals such as potassium and manganese.

Spring onions are a rich source of vitamins C and K. They also contain minerals such as potassium and small amounts of manganese. Oats provide nutrients such as manganese, phosphorus, and magnesium. Turmeric contains curcumin, which is known for its potential health benefits. Lime or lemon juice provides vitamin C and contains minerals such as potassium. The antioxidant content of this recipe comes from ingredients such as asparagus, sweet potatoes, and lime or lemon juice, all of which are known for their antioxidant properties. Oats, particularly beta-glucan, are rich in soluble fiber and contain B vitamins and minerals. Dietary fiber (DF) can be divided into soluble (pectins, gums, mucilage, and storage polysaccharides) and insoluble fiber (cellulose, hemicelluloses, lignin) based on water solubility. Soluble fiber stabilizes glucose and lipid metabolism, partly because of the increased viscosity of luminal contents. Soluble fiber provides short-chain fatty acids in the colon, which may benefit lipid metabolism and prevent cardiovascular disease. Vegetables in this recipe are a good source of vitamins, minerals, and polyphenols.

Mushroom Burger

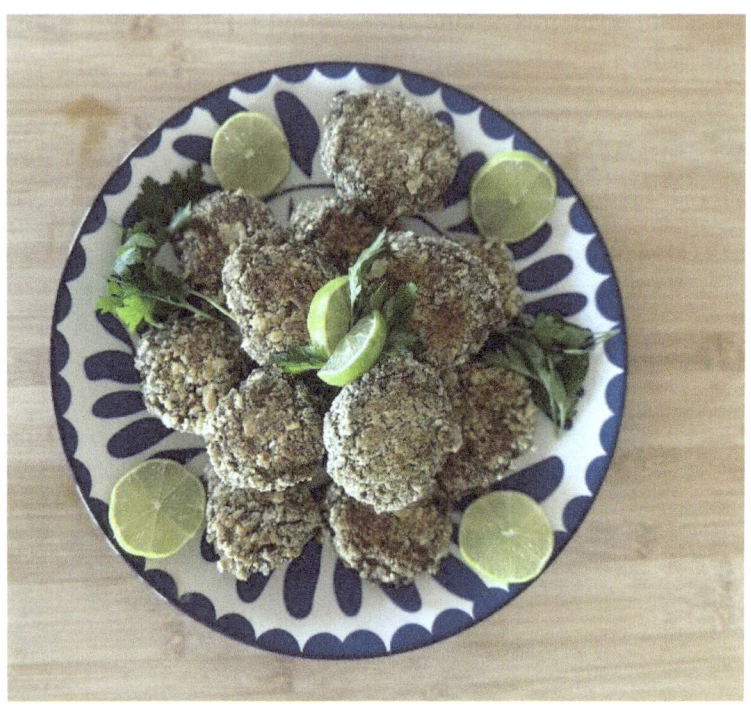

Total Preparation Time: 20-25 minutes
Total Cooking Time: 30-35 minutes
Serves: 4-6

Ingredients:
- ✓ 1 cup chopped portobello mushrooms or any type available (250 g / 8.8 oz.)
- ✓ ½ cup green lentils (100 g / 3.5 oz.)
- ✓ 1/2 cup diced onions (125 g / 4.4 oz.)
- ✓ 6 tablespoons good quality olive oil (60 g / 2.1 oz.)
- ✓ ½ cup chopped and roasted walnuts (125 g / 4.4 oz.)
- ✓ 2 tablespoons chives (6 g / 0.2 oz.)
- ✓ ½ cup chopped parsley (30 g / 1 oz.)
- ✓ 2 tablespoons garlic powder (20 g / 0.7 oz.)
- ✓ 1 teaspoon turmeric (3–5 g / 0.1 oz.)
- ✓ 1 teaspoon ground cumin seeds (3–5 g / 0.1 oz.)
- ✓ 1 teaspoon paprika (3–5 g / 0.1 oz.)
- ✓ 1 cup organic homemade breadcrumbs (from 2 slices of bread, 60 g / 2.1 oz.)
- ✓ ½ cup water or lemon juice to adjust the consistency (125 g/4 oz).

Recipe:
1. Add the green lentils and water to a small pan and cook for twenty minutes.
2. Once the green lentils are cooked, drain the water and set them aside.
3. Add four tablespoons of good-quality olive oil to a pan, then add the chopped mushrooms and onion.
4. Add all the chopped herbs and spices to the pan and let it simmer for a few minutes.
5. Once cooked, blend all the ingredients in a blender until smooth.

6. Scoop the mixture from the blender, then blend the walnuts and bread crumbs.
7. Then add the breadcrumb and walnut mix to the mushroom mixture and form it into a burger.
8. Pour two tablespoons of good-quality olive oil into the oven or air fryer.
9. Cook the burgers at 350°F for 20 minutes, or until they are golden brown.
10. Serve on an organic bun with a slice of onion, a slice of tomato, homemade salad dressing, and a green salad.

Homemade salad dressing (½ teaspoon Dijon mustard, three tablespoons virgin olive oil, lemon juice, salt and pepper, ½ teaspoon Italian herbs, all mixed together).

Total Nutritional Values of Mushroom Burger Recipe

Total Calories: 1,867 Kcal
Total Protein: 39g
Total Carbohydrates: 118g
Total Fat: 140g
Total Dietary Fiber: 26g

Mushrooms are a good source of beta-glucans and provide vitamins such as vitamin D (when exposed to sunlight), vitamin B3 (niacin), and small amounts of vitamins B5 (pantothenic acid) and B2 (riboflavin). They also contain essential minerals, including potassium, phosphorus, and selenium. Onions contain vitamins C and B6 (pyridoxine).

They also provide minerals such as potassium, as well as small amounts of manganese and copper. Good-quality olive oil (mainly monounsaturated fats) contains vitamins E and K. Chopped and roasted walnuts provide vitamins E and small amounts of B vitamins.

Walnuts also contain minerals such as magnesium, along with small amounts of potassium and zinc. Chives provide vitamins K and C, as well as minerals such as potassium, calcium, and iron. Parsley is rich in vitamin K and provides vitamins A and C, as well as minerals such as potassium, calcium, and iron. Garlic powder contains small amounts of vitamins C and B6 (pyridoxine). It also provides minerals, including manganese, along with small amounts of calcium and iron. Turmeric contains curcumin, which is also found in other recipes and is recognized for its potential health benefits. Cumin contains small amounts of vitamins, such as vitamin B1 (Thiamin), and minerals, including iron and manganese. Paprika contains various vitamins and minerals, including vitamins A and E. Bread crumbs may provide small amounts of vitamins, such as the B vitamins.

Eggplant Tofu Stew

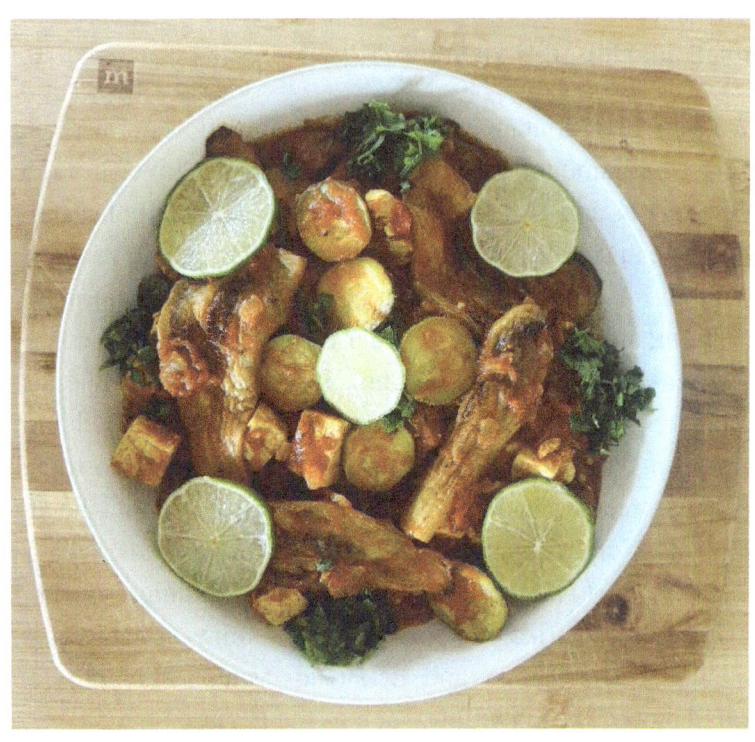

Total Preparation Time: 30-35 minutes
Total Cooking Time: 25-30 minutes
Serves: 4-6

Ingredients:
- ✓ 2 medium-sized eggplants (600 g / 21 oz.)
- ✓ 2 medium-sized zucchini (courgette) (400 g / 14 oz.)
- ✓ 1 cup organic tomato sauce (200 g / 7 oz) or six fresh organic tomatoes (400 g / 14 oz.)
- ✓ 1 tablespoon organic tomato puree (20 g / 0.7 oz.)
- ✓ 2 cloves garlic, minced (6 g / 0.2 oz.)
- ✓ ½ cup chopped organic tofu (100 g / 3.5 oz.)
- ✓ 1 medium-sized onion, chopped (150 g / 5.3 oz.)
- ✓ 3 medium-sized organic tomatoes, sliced (450 g / 16 oz.)
- ✓ 1 teaspoon turmeric (3–5 g / 0.1 oz.)
- ✓ 1 teaspoon curry powder (3–5 g / 0.1 oz.)
- ✓ 1 teaspoon cinnamon (3–5 g / 0.1 oz.)
- ✓ ½ teaspoon cayenne pepper (optional)
- ✓ ½ teaspoon cardamom
- ✓ 1–2 bay leaves
- ✓ Juice of 1–2 lemons
- ✓ ½ cup good-quality olive oil (120 g / 4.2 oz.)
- ✓ Salt and pepper to taste

Recipe:
1. Wash the eggplants and zucchini, then remove their skins.
2. Slice them lengthwise. Sprinkle salt on the eggplants to remove any bitterness.
3. Next, place the parchment paper in the oven and arrange the eggplants, zucchini, chopped onions, and tomato slices on it.

4. Add good-quality olive oil to the vegetables and cook at 350°F for 15-20 minutes, or until golden.
5. Pour some good-quality olive oil into a medium-sized pan, then add the minced garlic, spices, and tofu cubes.
6. Then add tomato puree and one cup of organic tomato sauce.
7. Then carefully transfer the vegetable slices from the oven to the pan and let all the ingredients cook together for 15-20 minutes over medium-low heat.
8. Add salt and pepper to taste, along with a squeeze of lemon juice.
9. This dish can be served on its own or with basmati rice and salad.

Total Nutritional Values of Eggplant Tofu Stew Recipe

Total Calories: 1565 Kcal
Total protein: 33g
Total carbohydrates: 130 g
Total fats: 125 g
Total Dietary Fiber: 41g

Eggplants provide vitamins such as vitamin K and small amounts of vitamin C and vitamin B6 (pyridoxine). They contain minerals like potassium and small amounts of manganese. Zucchini provides vitamins such as C and small amounts of B6 (pyridoxine). It contains minerals like potassium and small amounts of manganese. Tomatoes are a good source of vitamin C and provide vitamins A and K. They also contain minerals such as potassium and small amounts of manganese. Garlic contains small amounts of vitamins C and B6 (pyridoxine). It provides minerals such as manganese, along with small amounts of calcium and iron. Tofu is a good source of various B vitamins, including B1 (thiamin) and B2 (riboflavin). It contains essential minerals, including calcium, magnesium, and iron. Onions contain vitamins C and B6 (pyridoxine), as well as minerals such as potassium, small amounts of manganese, and copper. Tomatoes are a good source of vitamin C and provide vitamins A and K. They also contain minerals such as potassium, as well as small amounts of manganese and copper.

Turmeric contains curcumin, which is known for its potential health benefits. Curcumin, the primary bioactive compound in turmeric, is known for its potent anti-inflammatory properties. It may help reduce inflammation, which is linked to various chronic diseases. It is also known for its antioxidant properties and for neutralizing harmful free radicals. Antioxidants play a crucial role in protecting cells from oxidative damage and the effects of aging. The nutritional content of curry powder can vary based on its ingredients. It may contain small amounts of various vitamins and minerals. Cinnamon contains small amounts of vitamins and minerals, including manganese. Cayenne pepper is a source of vitamin A and small amounts of vitamin E. Olive oil (mainly healthy monounsaturated fats) contains vitamins E and K.

Herbal Nutty Pesto Spread

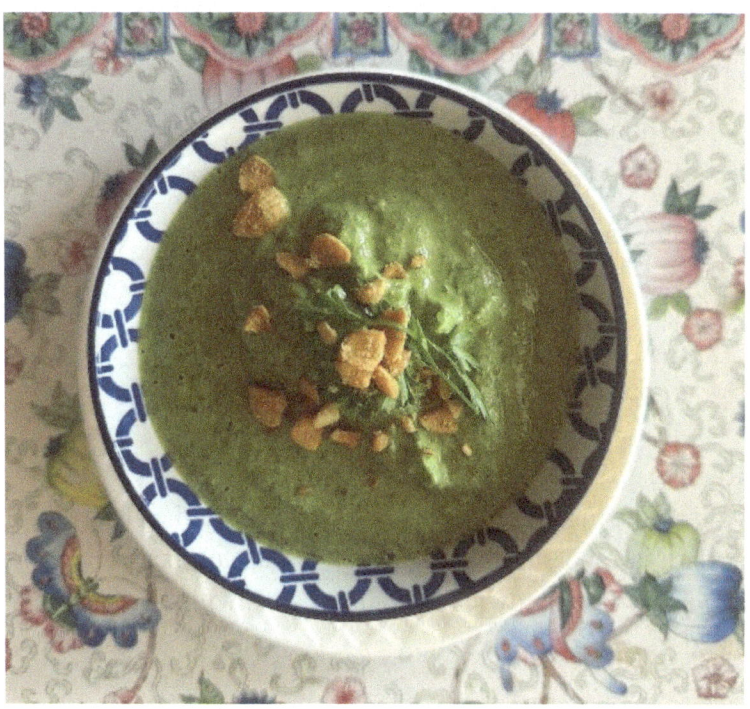

Total Preparation Time: 15-20 minutes
Total Cooking Time: No cooking required
Serves: 4

Ingredients:
- ✓ 1 cup chopped fresh organic parsley (60 g / 2.1 oz.)
- ✓ ½ cup of a mixture of raw, unsalted cashews, walnuts, and almonds (75 g / 2.6 oz.)
- ✓ 2 tablespoons of organic tahini (30 g / 1 oz.)
- ✓ 2 cloves garlic (6 g / 0.2 oz.)
- ✓ Juice of 2 lemons or limes, freshly squeezed (60 g / 2 oz.)
- ✓ 1 serrano pepper or hot sauce (10 g / 0.4 oz.)
- ✓ 1 teaspoon turmeric (3–5 g / 0.1 oz.)
- ✓ Water to adjust consistency
- ✓ Salt and pepper to taste

Recipe:

Add all the ingredients to the food processor, then transfer to a glass jar and store in the fridge for up to one week. You can use it as a sandwich spread or pair it with a green, leafy salad.

Total Nutritional Values of Herbal Nutty Pesto Spread

Total Calories: 582 Kcal
Total Carbohydrates: 42g
Total Protein: 19g
Total Fat: 44.4g
Total Dietary Fiber: 10 g

The antioxidant content in this recipe is primarily contributed by ingredients such as parsley (vitamin C), nuts (vitamin E and flavonoids), and turmeric (curcumin), all of which are known for their antioxidant properties. Parsley is a good source of vitamins K, C, and A. It also provides minerals, such as potassium, calcium, and iron. Parsley contains various polyphenols, including flavonoids and phenolic acids, such as apigenin and myricetin. Garlic contains small amounts of vitamins like vitamin C and vitamin B6 (Pyridoxine). It provides minerals such as manganese, along with small amounts of calcium and iron. Citrus fruits, such as lemons and limes, contain polyphenols, including flavonoids. They are excellent sources of vitamin C. They also provide small amounts of vitamin B6 (pyridoxine) and vitamin A. Lemons offer minerals like potassium and calcium. Nuts in this recipe are a good source of vitamin E and provide small amounts of B vitamins, such as riboflavin and niacin.

Nuts and seeds, including cashews, are rich in minerals such as magnesium, zinc, iron, and copper. Nuts, including walnuts and almonds, contain polyphenols, primarily flavonoids and phenolic acids. Serrano peppers contain polyphenols, including capsaicinoids, which give them their spicy flavor. Serrano peppers are a good source of vitamin C.

Serrano peppers provide minerals such as potassium. Turmeric in this recipe contains a bioactive compound, curcumin, a polyphenol with potential health benefits. Turmeric also contains small amounts of vitamins B6 (pyridoxine) and C, as well as minerals like manganese and iron. Tahini provides vitamins B1 (thiamine), B2 (riboflavin), B3 (niacin), B5 (pantothenic acid), B9 (folate), and vitamin E, as well as minerals such as calcium, magnesium, phosphorus, potassium, and zinc.

Hazelnut, Pumpkin Seed, and Herbal Tempeh Salad

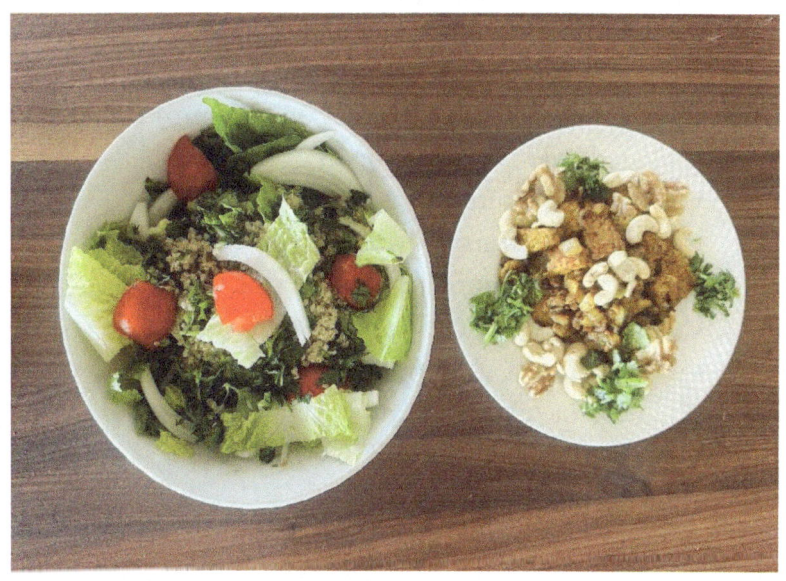

Preparation time: 15 minutes
Cooking time: 20 minutes
Serves: 4

Ingredients:
- ½ cup cooked quinoa (90g, 3.2 oz)
- 4 cups of mixed leaves or 140 g, 5.0oz.
- 1 medium-sized tomato, chopped, or 140g (5.0 oz).
- ½ English cucumber, cut into squares 150 g, 5.3 oz.
- ½ red onion, sliced or 75 g, or 2.6oz.
- ½ cup mixed herbs (parsley and cilantro) 10g, 0.3oz.
- ½ red onion, chopped or 75 g, or 2.6oz.
- ½ teaspoon turmeric 2.5g
- ½ teaspoon curry powder 2.5g
- ½ teaspoon paprika 2.5g
- ¼ cup olive oil or 54g, or 1.9oz.
- 3 oz tempeh, chopped 85g or 3.0 oz.
- ¼ cup hazelnuts, roughly chopped 30g or 1oz.
- ¼ cup pumpkin seeds 30g or 1oz.
- Salt and pepper to taste
- Salad dressing (1 teaspoon nutritional yeast, one tablespoon olive oil, one tablespoon apple cider vinegar, salt, and pepper to taste)

Recipe:
1. Rinse ½ cup of quinoa under cold water.
2. In a saucepan, combine the quinoa with 1 cup of water.
3. Bring to a boil, then reduce the heat to low, cover, and simmer for 15 minutes, until the quinoa is cooked and the water is absorbed.
4. Fluff with a fork and let it cool.
5. Wash and finely chop one cup of mixed herbs (parsley and cilantro).

6. Cut 3 oz of tempeh into small cubes or slices.
7. Chop half an onion and add it to a pan with a drizzle of olive oil.
8. Next, add the tempeh, herbs, spices, salt, and pepper, then cook the mixture for 5 minutes over medium heat.
9. Combine the mixed greens, cucumber, sliced onion, and tomatoes with the cooked quinoa and tempeh mixture in a large bowl.
10. In a dry pan over medium heat, toast ¼ cup each of hazelnuts and pumpkin seeds until lightly browned and fragrant, about 3-4 minutes.
11. Toast the nuts and seeds, then add them to the salad. If you don't have much time, just add the nuts without toasting them.

Dressing: In a small bowl, combine one tablespoon of olive oil, one tablespoon of apple cider vinegar, and 1 teaspoon of nutritional yeast. Season with salt and pepper to taste. Drizzle the dressing over the salad.

Total Nutritional Values Hazelnut and Pumpkin Seed Tempeh Salad

Total Calories: 1133 Kcal
Protein: 33 g
Carbohydrates: 36 g
Fat: 98 g
Total Fiber: 36 g

Cooked quinoa is a good source of protein, iron, magnesium, phosphorus, and zinc. Mixed herbs (parsley and cilantro) are a good source of calcium, iron, magnesium, and potassium. Tempeh is a good source of protein and contains B vitamins, including vitamin B2 (riboflavin), B3 (niacin), and B6 (pyridoxine), as well as minerals such as calcium, iron, magnesium, and zinc. Hazelnuts are an excellent source of magnesium, copper, iron, and zinc. Pumpkin seeds are an excellent source of magnesium, iron, and zinc. Nutritional yeast is a good source of B vitamins, iron, and zinc. This salad offers a rich source of vitamins, including A, C, E, and K, as well as several B vitamins. It is a good source of essential minerals, including magnesium, iron, calcium, and zinc. The polyphenol content of pumpkin seeds, including flavonoids, and of hazelnuts and olive oil, including ellagic acid, as well as oleuropein, hydroxytyrosol, and tyrosol, exhibits antioxidant properties. Polyphenols are found in herbs, and apigenin and quercetin are found in onions. This nutrient-dense salad offers a balanced combination of essential vitamins, minerals, and polyphenols, making it a healthful addition to your diet.

Homemade Berry Ice Cream

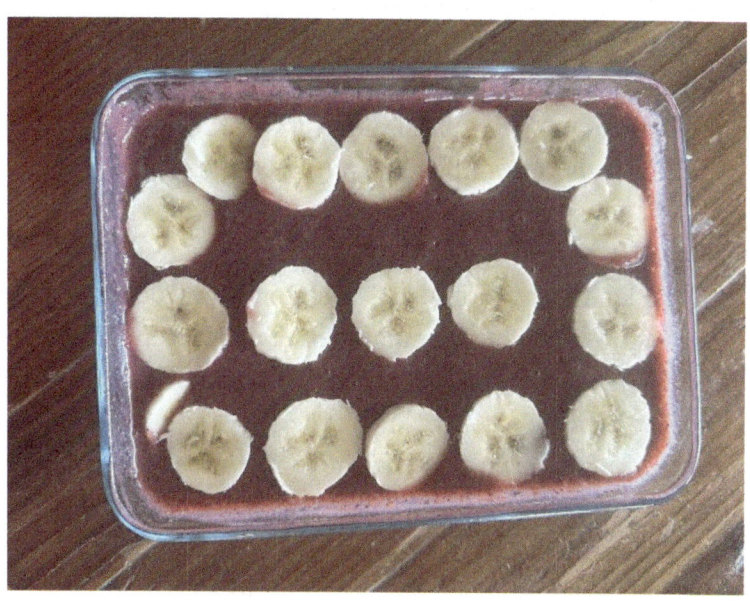

Total Preparation Time: 10-15 minutes
Freezing Time: 2-3 hours
Serves: 2-3

Ingredients:
- ✓ 1 cup organic frozen strawberries (150 g / 5.3 oz)
- ✓ 1 cup organic raspberries (125 g / 4.4 oz)
- ✓ 8 Medjool dates, deseeded (200 g / 7 oz)
- ✓ 1 cup organic almond milk (240 g / 8.5 oz)
- ✓ Slices of 1 banana for decoration (120 g / 4.2 oz)
- ✓ 1 teaspoon vanilla extract (5 g / 0.2 oz)

Recipe:
1. Blend the berries, dates, almond milk, and vanilla extract in a blender until smooth and creamy.
2. Add the milk gradually to achieve a smooth consistency.
3. Then, pour the mixture into a Pyrex container. Then slice a banana and arrange the slices on top to create a banana layer.
4. Place the lid on and freeze for 2 to 3 hours.

Total Nutritional Values of Homemade Berry Ice Cream

Total Calories: 816 Kcal
Total Protein: 7.5g
Total Carbohydrates: 204g
Total Fat: 3.5g
Total Dietary Fiber: 28g

As mentioned earlier, berries contain polyphenols and vitamin C, making them excellent sources of antioxidants. Antioxidants are compounds that help neutralize free radicals in the body, which can contribute to oxidative stress. While specific antioxidant values are not provided here, berries are a good source of vitamins, minerals, and phytochemicals with antioxidant properties.

Fruit Salad With Homemade Carrot Jam and Alternative Cream

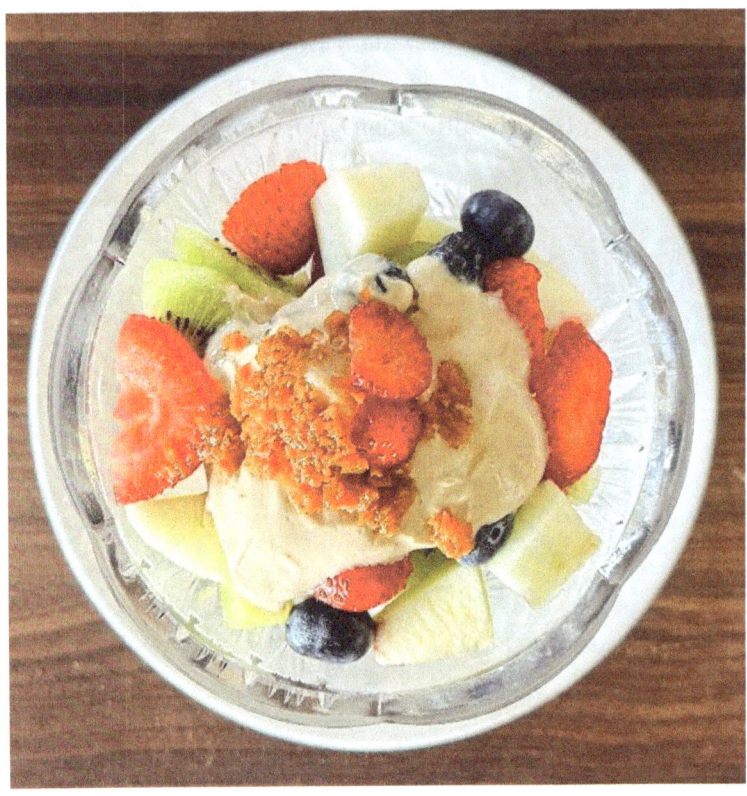

Preparation Time: 10-15 minutes
Cooking Time: No cooking is required for the fruit salad; allow time to make the Carrot Jam.
Serves: 1

Ingredients:
- ✓ 1 whole kiwi, sliced (100 g / 3.5 oz)
- ✓ 1 whole apple, sliced (200 g / 7 oz)
- ✓ 1 orange, sliced (200 g / 7 oz)
- ✓ 1/2 cup strawberries (75 g / 2.6 oz)
- ✓ 1/2 cup blueberries (75 g / 2.6 oz)

Recipe:

Place the sliced fruits and berries in a bowl. It is a good idea to make jam and an alternative to cream ahead of time, then store them in a glass jar in the fridge for a week or so, to top the fruit salad if one wishes.

The recipe for jam and cream is indicated below.

Total Nutritional Values for the Fruit Salad Recipe

Total Calories: 265 Kcal
Total Carbohydrates: 67g
Total Protein: 3g
Total Fat: 1g
Total Dietary Fiber: 12g

Kiwi is rich in vitamin C and provides small amounts of vitamins A and E, as well as vitamin K. It contains minerals such as potassium, along with small amounts of calcium and magnesium. Apples provide vitamin C and small amounts of vitamins A and B6 (pyridoxine). They contain minerals such as potassium, along with small amounts of calcium and magnesium. Apples contain antioxidants like quercetin. Oranges are a rich source of vitamin C and provide vitamins A and B6 (pyridoxine). They contain minerals such as potassium, along with small amounts of calcium and magnesium. Oranges are renowned for their high antioxidant content, which includes vitamin C and flavonoids.

Strawberries are rich in vitamin C and provide small amounts of vitamins A and K. They also contain essential minerals such as potassium, calcium, and magnesium. Strawberries are renowned for their high antioxidant content, which includes vitamin C and anthocyanins.

Blueberries are a good source of vitamin C and also contain vitamins K and small amounts of vitamin A. They contain essential minerals, including potassium, calcium, and magnesium. Blueberries are also rich in fiber. Fruits, in general, are rich sources of antioxidants, particularly vitamin C and various phytochemicals, which help protect cells from oxidative damage.

Kiwi is a good source of fiber. It is rich in vitamin C, providing more than the daily recommended intake. They also contain vitamins K and E, as well as potassium and other essential nutrients.

Apples are an excellent source of fiber. They contain vitamin C and small amounts of vitamin A, potassium, and vitamin B6 (pyridoxine).

Oranges are rich in fiber and an excellent source of vitamin C, providing potassium, folate, and vitamin A. Strawberries are rich in vitamin C and manganese, and they also provide small amounts of other vitamins and minerals. Blueberries are renowned for their high anthocyanin and antioxidant content, which includes vitamins C and K, as well as manganese.

Carrot Jam

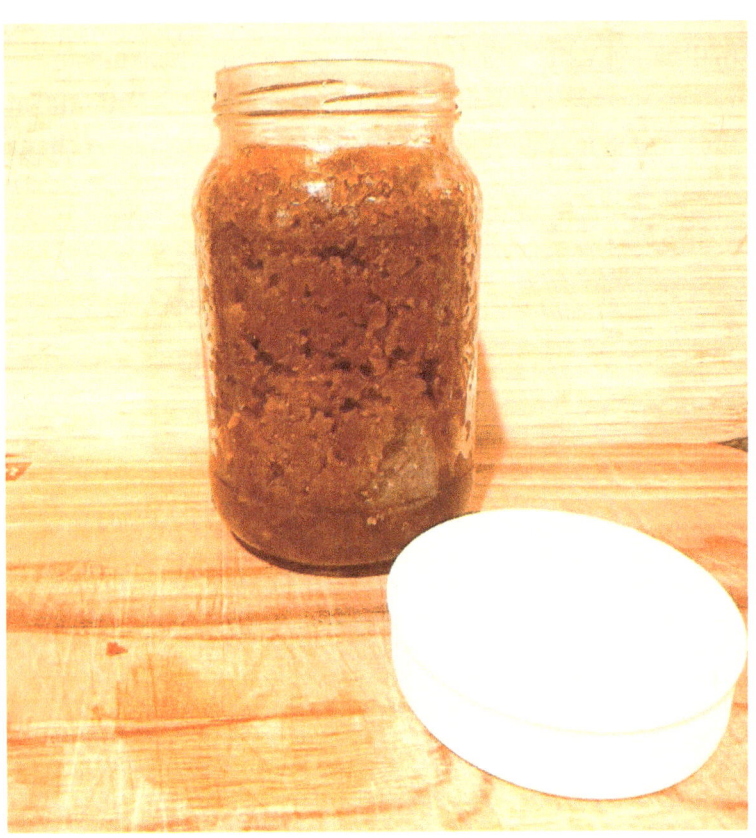

Total Preparation Time: 30 minutes
Total Cooking Time: 35-40 minutes
Serves: 4-6

Ingredients:
- ✓ 1 lb. or 2 cups organic carrots, grated (450 g / 16 oz)
- ✓ 1/2 cup of water (120 ml / 120 g / 4.2 oz)
- ✓ Coconut sugar (200 g / 7 oz)
- ✓ 1 teaspoon vanilla extract (5 g / 0.2 oz)
- ✓ 2 teaspoons cardamom (8–10 g / 0.4 oz)
- ✓ 1 teaspoon fresh lemon juice (5 g / 0.2 oz)

Recipe:
1. Allow the grated carrot to cook over a low flame, adding water and stirring every 5 minutes for the first 15 minutes.
2. Then add the remaining ingredients.
3. Cook over a low flame, stirring continuously with a wooden spoon. This process may take some time.
4. When the water has evaporated, add the coconut sugar. If you're using honey, add it at the end.
5. The jam is ready when a slight glaze forms on the carrots, and all the water has evaporated.

Please note that this recipe is low in sugar; therefore, the jam should be stored in the refrigerator and used within a few days. The jam can be stored in sterilized jars and sealed tightly. It can be stored in the fridge for up to a week and used for sweet treats, such as breakfast jam on toast, or added to a fruit salad as a dessert.

Total Nutritional Values for the Carrot Jam Recipe

> Total Calories: 898 Kcal (for coconut sugar) or 1,110 Kcal (for honey)
> Total Carbohydrates: 233g (for coconut sugar) or 317g (for honey)
> Total Protein: 6g
> Total Fat: 1g
> Total Dietary Fiber: 9g

Carrots are a rich source of vitamin A (beta-carotene) and provide vitamins such as vitamin K, as well as small amounts of vitamin C and vitamin B6 (pyridoxine). They contain minerals such as potassium, along with small amounts of calcium and iron. Cardamom contains small amounts of various vitamins and minerals. Lemon juice is a good source of vitamin C.

Ingredients such as carrots (a source of beta-carotene) primarily contribute to the recipe's antioxidant content. Cardamom may have a calming effect, helping to reduce stress and anxiety. It is used in aromatherapy for its mood-enhancing properties. Lemon juice contains vitamin C and other antioxidants. Honey and coconut sugar may also contain antioxidants.

Embrace The Young You

Alternative to Cream

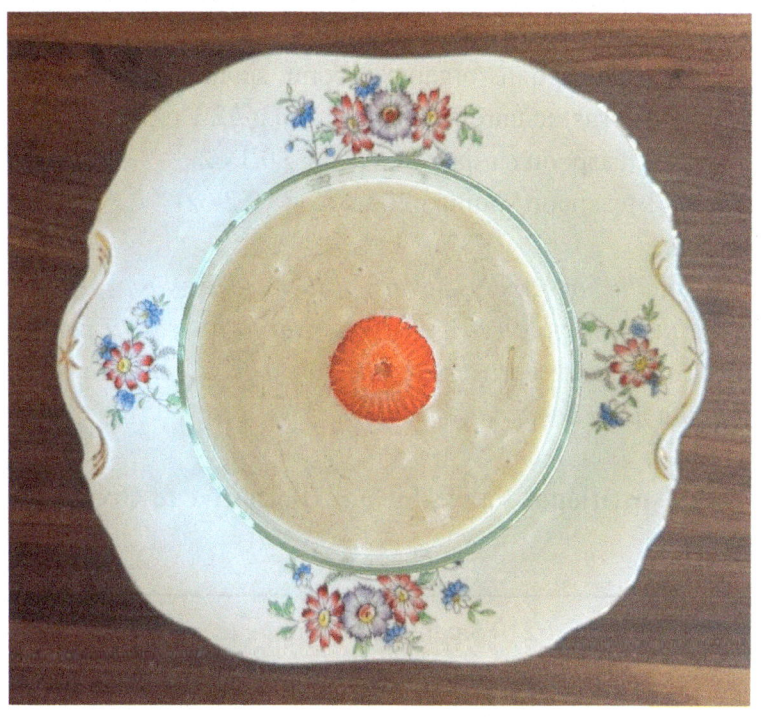

Total Preparation Time: 10-15 minutes
Total Cooking Time: 15-20 minutes
Serves: 4-6

Ingredients:
- ✓ 3 tablespoons Greek non-fat yogurt or non-dairy coconut yogurt (45 g / 1.6 oz)
- ✓ 3 tablespoons organic coconut sugar (45 g / 1.6 oz) or organic unrefined honey (60 g / 2.1 oz)
- ✓ 1 teaspoon cardamom (2–5 g / 0.1 oz)
- ✓ 1 teaspoon vanilla extract (5 g / 0.2 oz)

Recipe:
Mix all the ingredients, transfer them to a glass jar, and store the jar in the refrigerator for up to a week. It can be used as an alternative to cream on a fruit salad or as a topping for a homemade dessert.

Total Nutritional Values for an Alternative to Cream Recipe

Total Calories: 210 Kcal (for coconut sugar) or 222 Kcal (for honey)
Total Carbohydrates: 48g (for coconut sugar) or 55g (for honey)
Total Protein: 3g
Total Fat: 0g
Total Dietary Fiber: 0g

Yogurt is a good source of protein and is lower in fat than cream. Add vanilla, cardamom, and honey to any dessert for an extra layer of creaminess, richness, and flavor. Vanilla and cardamom are both anti-inflammatory and can help with digestion. Honey contains various phenolic acids, including gallic acid, caffeic acid, ferulic acid, and p-coumaric acid. These compounds have antioxidant and anti-inflammatory effects. They also contribute to the overall phenolic content of honey. Ellagic acid is another phenolic compound found in some types of honey. It has antioxidant properties and may help protect cells from oxidative damage. Some honey varieties contain cinnamic acid derivatives, including p-coumaric and caffeic acids. These compounds are recognized for their potential health benefits, including anti-inflammatory and antioxidant effects. Chrysin is a flavone found in honey. It has antioxidant properties and may offer health benefits, including anti-anxiety and anti-inflammatory effects. Pinocembrin is a flavanone found in honey, particularly in propolis (a resinous substance bees make). It has antioxidant properties and may have antimicrobial effects.

These phenolic compounds contribute to honey's distinctive flavor and aroma and are also responsible for its potential health benefits. However, the specific types and amounts of phenolic compounds can vary based on factors such as the honey's floral source and processing. In general, darker honey varieties contain higher levels of phenolic compounds than lighter ones.

Vegan option: Use coconut or soy yogurt, add coconut or date sugar for sweetness, and follow the rest of the recipe.

Embrace The Young You

Coconut, Oat, Banana Nut Cookies

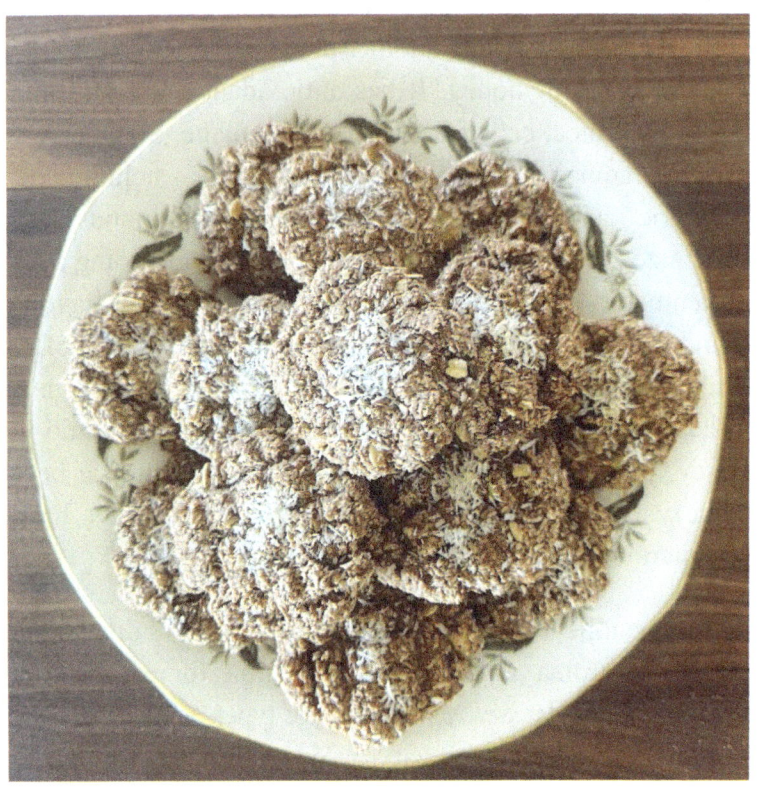

Total Preparation Time: 15 minutes
Total Cooking Time: 15-20 minutes
Serves: 12-16

Ingredients:
- ✓ 250 g or 1 cup organic coconut flakes (250 g / 8.8 oz.)
- ✓ 2 teaspoons organic cocoa powder (6–10 g / 0.2 oz.)
- ✓ 1 tablespoon homemade nut paste (15–20 g / 0.7 oz.)
- ✓ 2 medium-sized ripe bananas (300 g / 10.5 oz.)
- ✓ 2 cups organic oats, ground into flour (500 g / 17.6 oz.)
- ✓ 1 tablespoon good quality olive oil (15 g / 0.5 oz.)
- ✓ Pinch of salt
- ✓ 1 teaspoon lemon zest (5 g/ 0.1 oz.)
- ✓ 1 teaspoon baking powder (5 g / 0.2 oz.)
- ✓ 100 ml coconut water (100 g / 3.5 oz.)

Recipe:
1. In a medium-sized Pyrex bowl, mash two ripe bananas. Add a tablespoon each of homemade nut paste (see recipe below) and coconut water.
2. Add two teaspoons of cocoa powder.
3. Blend the organic oat grits into a flour-like consistency and add them to the wet ingredients.
4. Add a teaspoon each of baking powder, lemon zest, and vanilla.
5. Add coconut flakes and mix well.
6. Make small balls, place them on an oven tray, and press them into round cookies.
7. Bake at 350°F for 15-20 minutes, or until the cookies are golden brown on the outside.

Total Nutritional Values for The Coconut, Oat, Banana Nut Cookies Recipe

Calories: 1887 Kcal
Protein: 60.6g
Fat: 104.8g
Carbohydrates: 221.6g
Fiber: 47.7g

Mixed Nut Paste

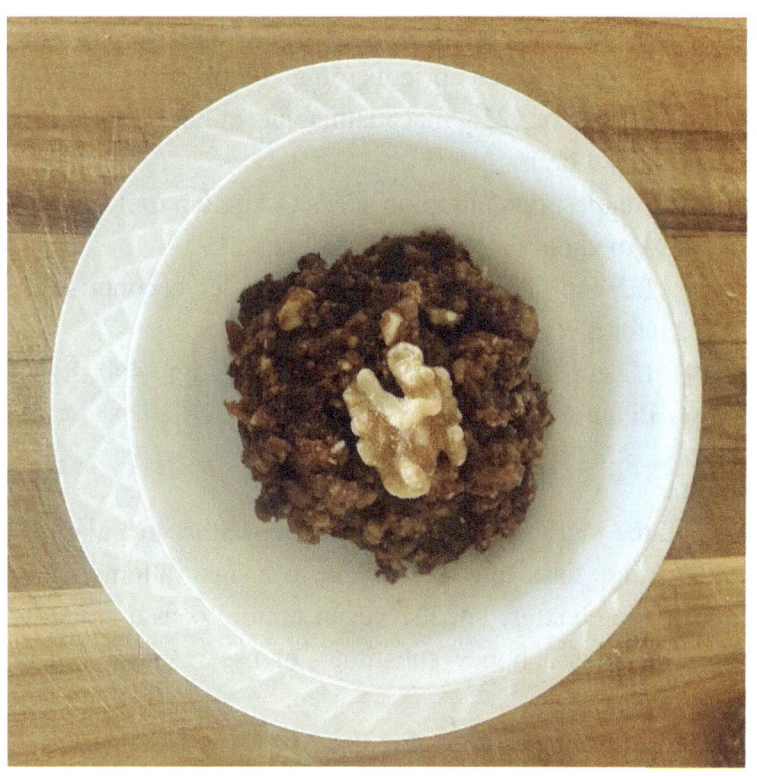

Preparation Time: 15 Minutes
Cooking Time: None
Serving: 6 portions

Ingredients:
- ✓ 1/2 tablespoon organic cocoa powder (6 g / 0.2 oz.)
- ✓ 4 organic dried apricots (60 g / 2.1 oz.)
- ✓ 1/2 cup or 125 g macadamia nuts or hazelnuts (125 g or 4.4 oz.)
- ✓ 1 tablespoon pumpkin seeds (15 g / 0.5 oz.)
- ✓ 4 medjool dates (100 g / 3.5 oz.)
- ✓ 1/2 cup (125 g) unrefined honey or coconut sugar (for a vegan option, 170 g/6 oz).
- ✓ 1/2 cup or 125 ml coconut water (125 g / 4.4 oz.)
- ✓ Pinch of sea salt

Recipe:
Mix all the ingredients in a food blender. Store in a glass jar in the fridge for a few weeks. Use as a sugar alternative in homemade cookies. For the vegan option, consider adding more dates as a honey substitute, or use maple syrup or coconut sugar.

Total Nutritional Values for the Nut Paste Recipe

Total Calories: 1820 Kcal
Total Protein: 20.7 g
Carbohydrates: 243.3g
Fat: 103.7 g
Fiber: 26.4

Nut Cookie Pastry

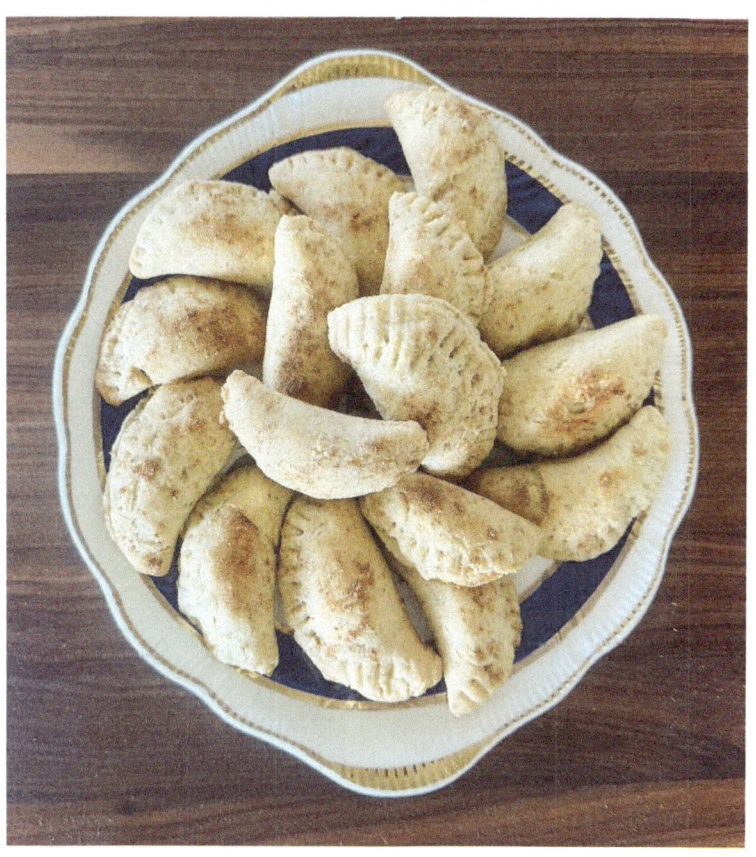

Total Preparation Time: 30 minutes
Total Cooking Time: 40-45 minutes
Serves: 16 -20 cookie portions

Ingredients:
- ✓ 3 cups organic flour (360 g / 12.7 oz.)
- ✓ 1 teaspoon baking powder (5 g / 0.2 oz.)
- ✓ 1 cup of good-quality olive oil (240 g / 8.5 oz.)
- ✓ 1 cup organic yogurt (240 g / 8.5 oz.)
- ✓ 1 organic egg (50 g / 1.8 oz., average size)
- ✓ 1/2 cup of honey or maple syrup (for vegan option)
  - Honey: (170 g / 6 oz.)
  - Maple syrup: (160 g / 5.6 oz.)
- ✓ 3 teaspoons cardamom (15 g / 0.5 oz.)
- ✓ 2 cups walnuts (200 g / 7 oz.)
- ✓ 1 teaspoon cinnamon (2–5 g / 0.1 oz.)
- ✓ 2 teaspoons rose water (10 g / 0.4 oz.)
- ✓ 1 cup dried mulberries (instead of sugar, 150 g / 5.3 oz.)

Recipe:
1. Mix the flour, baking powder, oil, yogurt, honey, and egg in a large bowl.
2. Mix all the ingredients thoroughly to form a dough. Allow the dough to rest in the refrigerator for at least an hour.
3. Meanwhile, put two cups of walnuts and one cup of *dried mulberries in a food processor to sweeten the walnuts.
4. Grind the walnuts and dried berries. You can use a mixture of nuts, such as walnuts, pistachios, and

almonds, if you prefer. Add the cardamom and cinnamon to the ground mixture.
5. Once the dough has rested, roll it out with a rolling pin. Then, using a cup as a circular mold, cut small circles from the rolled-out dough.
6. Place a teaspoon of the nut mixture in the center. Fold the dough into a crescent shape, ensuring the nut mixture is centered. Press the ends with a fork to seal the dough well.
7. Then preheat the oven to 350°F and bake the batch of Nut Cookie Pastry for 15-20 minutes, or until it is slightly golden.
8. Allow them to cool. One can sprinkle more cardamom and cinnamon on the Nut cookie pastries instead of sugar.

If dried mulberry is unavailable, add half a cup of coconut sugar instead of ordinary sugar for sweetness.

Vegan Option

One can use soy yogurt instead of egg and maple syrup or coconut sugar as a sweetener. Follow the recipe mentioned above and enjoy the nut pastry with tea or coffee. These nut pastries can be stored in the freezer in a container for freshness.

Total Nutritional Values for the Entire Nut Cookie Pastry Recipe

Calories: 5200 kcal
Protein: 104 g
Fat: 330 g
Carbohydrates: 540 g
Fiber: 47g

Blueberry and Banana Scones

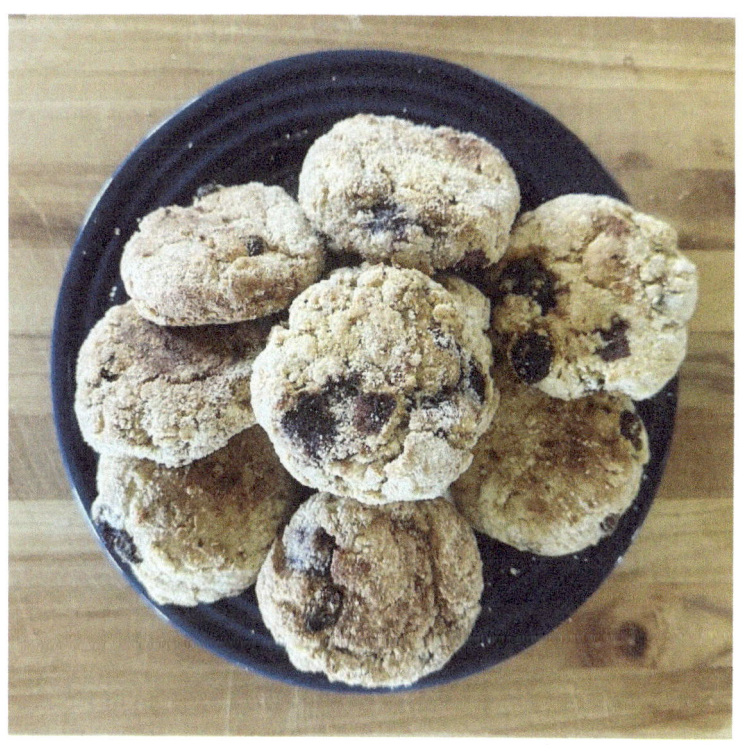

Preparation Time: 15 Minutes
Cooking Time: 30 Minutes
Serves: 8-10

Ingredients:
- ✓ 2 cups organic flour (240 g / 8.5 oz.)
- ✓ 2 cups almond flour (200 g / 7 oz.)
- ✓ 2 teaspoons cardamom (4 g / 0.1 oz.)
- ✓ 1 teaspoon vanilla extract (5 g / 0.2 oz.)
- ✓ 1 teaspoon baking powder (5 g / 0.2 oz.)
- ✓ 1 teaspoon bicarbonate of soda (baking soda) (5 g / 0.2 oz.)
- ✓ 4 tablespoons olive oil (60 g / 2.1 oz.)
- ✓ 4 tablespoons coconut milk (60 g / 2.1 oz.)
- ✓ 1/2 cup blueberries (50 g / 1.5 oz.)
- ✓ 1 ½ bananas, mashed (200 g / 7 oz.)
- ✓ 2 tablespoons raisins (30 g / 1 oz.)
- ✓ 2 tablespoons honey (30 g / 1 oz.) or maple syrup (for a vegan alternative, 30 g / 1 oz.)
- ✓ 1 teaspoon lemon zest (2–5 g/ 0.1 oz.)

Recipe:
1. Preheat your oven to 375°F (190°C) and line a baking sheet with parchment paper.
2. In a large mixing bowl, combine the organic flour, almond flour, cardamom, baking powder, and baking soda.
3. Add the olive oil and vanilla extract to the dry ingredients and mix until the mixture resembles coarse crumbs.
4. Gradually stir in the coconut milk, then add the blueberries, mashed bananas, raisins, and honey or

maple syrup until well combined and the mixture resembles a dough.
5. Transfer the dough to a lightly floured surface and knead until smooth. Pat the dough into a 1-inch-thick circle, then use a knife or pastry cutter to cut it into eight wedges.
6. Place the scones on the prepared baking sheet, leaving space between them.
7. Bake in the oven for 18-20 minutes, or until the scones are golden brown and cooked through.
8. Remove the scones from the oven and let them cool on the baking sheet for a few minutes. Then transfer them to a wire rack to cool completely.
9. Serve the blueberry and banana scones warm or at room temperature, and enjoy them with a cup of tea or coffee!

Total Nutrition Values of The Blueberry and Banana Scones Recipe

Calories: 2850 Kcal
Protein: 85g
Total Carbohydrates: 360g
Total Fat: 130g
Dietary Fiber: 40g

Gluten-free Banana Cookies

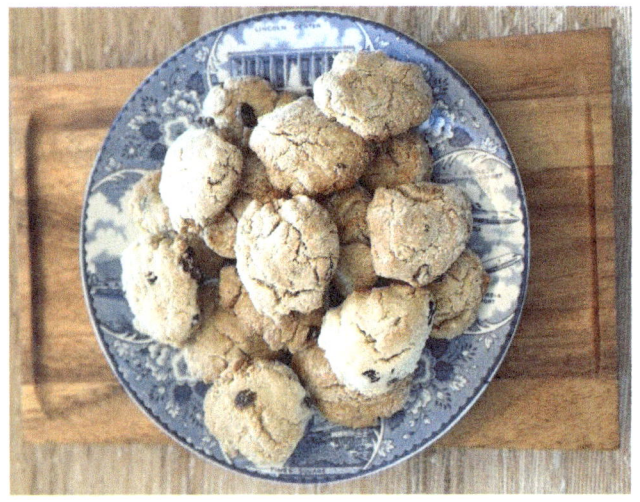

Total Preparation Time: 15 minutes
Total Cooking Time: 20-25 minutes
Serves: 15

Ingredients:
- ✓ 1 ripe banana (120 g / 4.2 oz.)
- ✓ 1/2 cup yogurt (use soy yogurt for vegan option, 120 g / 4.2 oz.)
- ✓ 2 cups gluten-free organic rolled oats (200 g / 7 oz.)
- ✓ 2 cups almond flour (200 g / 7 oz.)
- ✓ 4 tablespoons honey or date syrup (for vegan option), Honey: (80 g / 2.8 oz), Date syrup: (80 g / 2.8 oz.)
- ✓ ¼ cup chopped nuts (walnuts, pecans, etc., 30 g / 1 oz.)
- ✓ ¼ cup raisins (40 g / 1.4 oz.)
- ✓ 1 teaspoon ground cinnamon (2–5 g / 0.1 oz.)
- ✓ 1 teaspoon ground cardamom (2 g / 0.1 oz.)
- ✓ 4 tablespoons olive oil (60 g / 2.1 oz.)
- ✓ 1 teaspoon baking powder (5 g / 0.2 oz.)
- ✓ ½ tablespoon baking soda (7 g / 0.5 oz.)
- ✓ 1 teaspoon lemon zest (2–5 g/ 0.1 oz.)
- ✓ ¼ teaspoon vanilla extract
- ✓ Pinch of salt

Recipe:
1. Preheat your oven to 350°F (175°C).
2. Line a baking sheet with parchment paper or lightly grease it. In a mixing bowl, mash the ripe bananas until smooth.
3. Grind the rolled oats in a food processor until they reach a flour-like consistency.

4. Add the gluten-free rolled oats, almond flour, yogurt, olive oil, chopped nuts, raisins, ground cinnamon, vanilla extract, cardamom, lemon zest, and a pinch of salt to the mashed bananas.
5. Stir well until all ingredients are evenly mixed.
6. Using a spoon or an ice cream scoop, drop dollops of the cookie dough onto the prepared baking sheet, leaving space between each scone.
7. Use the back of the spoon or your fingers to slightly flatten each cookie, as they won't spread much during baking.
8. Bake in the oven for 12-15 minutes, or until the cookies are golden brown around the edges. Once baked, remove the cookies from the oven and let them cool on the baking sheet for a few minutes.
9. Transfer the cookies to a wire rack to cool completely before serving.

You can customize the recipe by adding mixed nuts, chocolate chips, coconut flakes, or dried fruit.

Total Nutritional Values of The Gluten-Free Banana Cookies Recipe

Calories:	3061 Kcal
Protein:	81.8 g
Carbohydrates:	288.6g
Fat:	201.7g
Fiber:	45.1g

Gluten-Free Blueberry and Raisin Scones

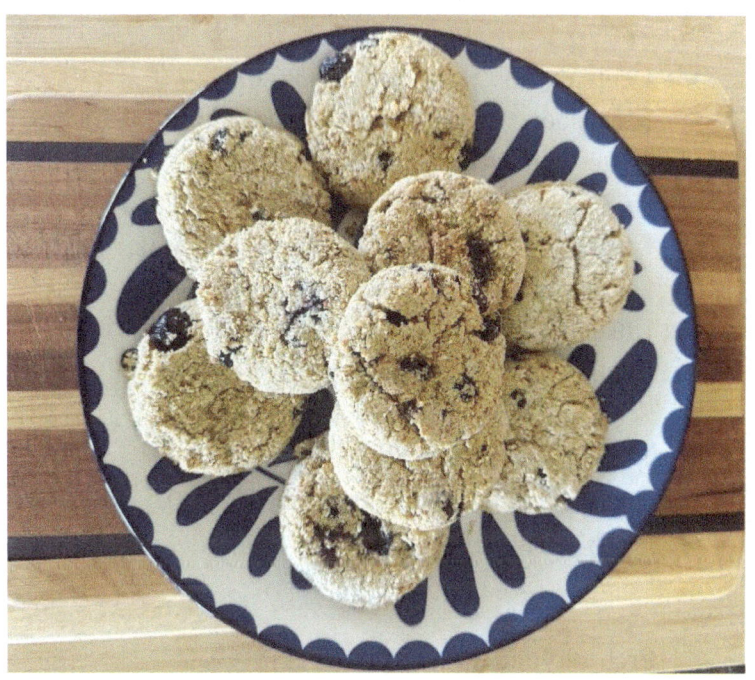

Total Preparation Time: 20 minutes
Total Cooking Time: 20-25 minutes
Serves: 12

Ingredients:
- ✓ 1 cup blueberries (fresh or frozen, 150 g / 5.3 oz.)
- ✓ ½ cup raisins (75 g / 2.6 oz.)
- ✓ 2 cups gluten-free rolled oats (ground into flour, 200 g / 7 oz.)
- ✓ 1 cup almond flour (100 g / 3.5 oz.)
- ✓ 1 teaspoon vanilla extract (5 g / 0.2 oz.)
- ✓ 1 cup yogurt (for vegan option, use soy yogurt, 240 g / 8.5 oz.)
- ✓ 1 teaspoon ground cardamom (2 g / 0.1 oz.)
- ✓ 1 teaspoon ground cinnamon (2 g / 0.1 oz.)
- ✓ 1 teaspoon lemon zest (2 g/ 0.1 oz.)
- ✓ 1 teaspoon baking powder (5 g / 0.2 oz.)
- ✓ ½ teaspoon baking soda (2.5 g / 0.1 oz.)/
- ✓ 4 tablespoons olive oil (60 g / 2.1 oz.)
- ✓ ¼ cup coconut flakes (optional, 15 g / 0.5 oz.)
- ✓ Pinch of salt

Recipe:
1. Preheat your oven to 350°F (175°C).
2. Line a baking sheet with parchment paper or lightly grease it. Combine the ground rolled oats, almond flour, baking powder, baking soda, ground cardamom, cinnamon, lemon zest, and a pinch of salt in a mixing bowl.
3. Mix well to combine.
4. Whisk together the yogurt, olive oil, and vanilla extract in another bowl until smooth.

5. Gradually add the wet ingredients to the dry ingredients, stirring until a dough forms.
6. Gently fold the blueberries, raisins, and coconut flakes (if using) into the dough until evenly distributed. Transfer the dough to a lightly floured surface.
7. Shape it into a circle or rectangle, 1 inch thick.
8. Cut the dough into eight wedges or squares using a knife or pastry cutter.
9. Place the scones on the prepared baking sheet, leaving some space between them.
10. Bake in the oven for 18-20 minutes, or until the scones are golden brown and cooked through.
11. Once baked, remove the scones from the oven and allow them to cool slightly on the baking sheet before transferring them to a wire rack to finish cooling.

Total Nutritional Values of The Gluten-Free Blueberry and Raisin Scones Recipe

Total Calories: 2283 Kcal
Protein: 48.1g
Carbohydrates: 266g
Fat: 146.5g
Fiber: 37g

Homemade Organic Flat Sourdough Bread

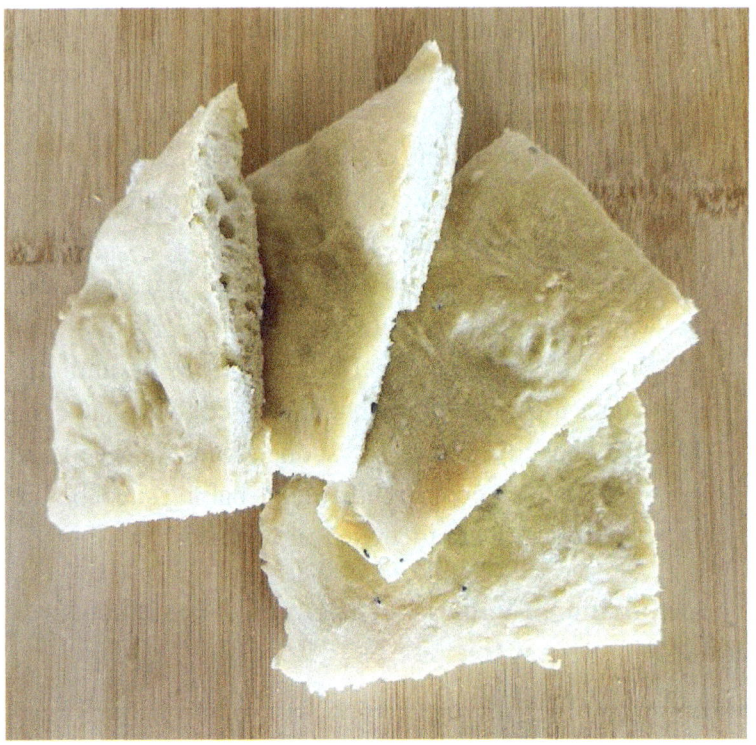

Preparation Time: 15 minutes
Resting Time: 2-3 hours
Serves: 10-12 slices

Ingredients:
- ✓ 2 cups organic flour (240 g / 8.5 oz.)
- ✓ 1 cup sourdough starter (240 g / 8.5 oz.; weight can vary)
- ✓ 1 teaspoon salt (5 g / 0.2 oz.)
- ✓ 1 tablespoon olive oil (15 g / 0.5 oz.)
- ✓ 1 tablespoon black seeds (nigella seeds, 10-15 g / 0.4 oz.)
- ✓ 1 teaspoon turmeric powder (2-5 g / 0.1 oz.)
- ✓ 1 teaspoon garlic powder (2-5 g / 0.1 oz.)
- ✓ 1 tablespoon sesame seeds (10-15 g / 0.4 oz.)
- ✓ Water (as needed): The amount required can vary, but typically around ½ to 1 cup (120-240 ml) is enough to achieve the right dough consistency.

Recipe:
1. Combine the organic bread flour, salt, turmeric powder, garlic powder, and black seeds in a large mixing bowl. Mix thoroughly to evenly distribute the dry ingredients.
2. Add the sourdough starter and olive oil to the dry ingredients. Mix the dough, gradually adding water until it is slightly sticky. The exact amount of water may vary based on the flour and the hydration level of your sourdough starter.
3. Once the dough comes together, transfer it to a lightly floured surface and knead it for 8-10 minutes, or until smooth and elastic.
4. Place the dough in a lightly oiled bowl, cover it with a clean kitchen towel or plastic wrap, and let it rise

in a warm place for 4-6 hours, or until it doubles in size.
5. This fermentation time allows the sourdough to develop flavor and rise.
6. After the dough has doubled in size, gently deflate it and shape it into a loaf.
7. You can shape it into a round or flat shape for flat bread.
8. Place the dough on a parchment-lined baking sheet and roll it into a flat shape with a rolling pin, or place it in a lightly greased loaf pan or Dutch oven. Cover with a clean kitchen towel and let it rise for 2-4 hours, or until it has doubled in size.
9. Preheat your oven to 425°F (220°C). If desired, slash the top of the bread with a sharp knife to create decorative patterns.
10. Bake the bread for 35 minutes until it is golden on top.
11. Once baked, remove the bread from the oven and let it cool on a wire rack before slicing and serving.

Total Nutritional Values of Sourdough Bread:

Total Calories: 1365 Kcal
Total Protein: 42g
Total Carbohydrates: 71g
Total Fat: 17g
Total Fiber: 6g

Homemade Pizza with Tofu Cheese

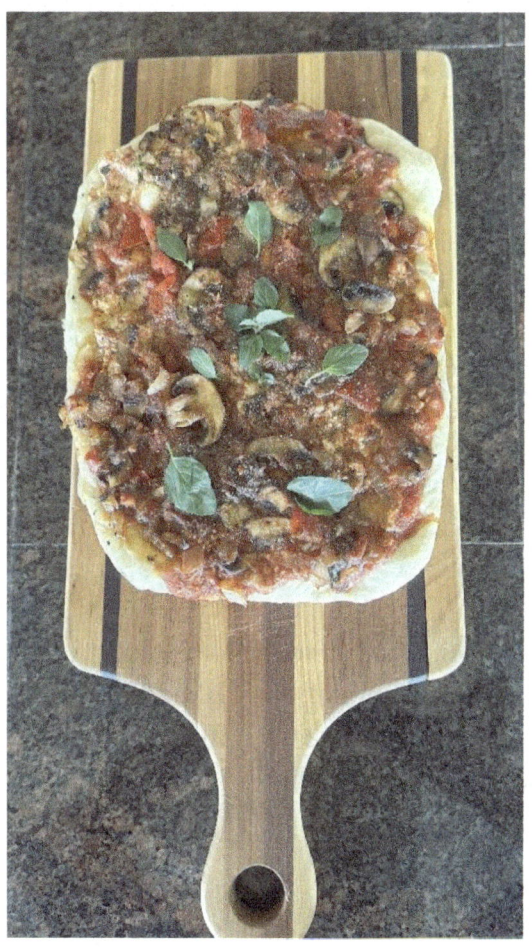

Preparation Time: 1-2 hours
Cooking Time: 30 minutes
Serves: 5

For the pizza dough:
Ingredients:
- ✓ 2 cups organic all-purpose flour
- ✓ 1 teaspoon salt
- ✓ 1 teaspoon organic honey (or maple syrup for a vegan option)
- ✓ 1 tablespoon olive oil
- ✓ 1 cup lukewarm water
- ✓ 2 ¼ teaspoons active dry yeast

For the toppings:
- ✓ 1 cup organic tomato sauce (240 g or 8.5 oz.)
- ✓ 1 cup crumbled organic tofu
- ✓ 1 cup crushed cashew nuts (120 g or 4 oz.)
- ✓ 1 teaspoon nutritional yeast (5 g or 0.1 oz.)
- ✓ 1 cup sliced tomatoes (150 g or 5.3 oz.)
- ✓ ½ cup thinly sliced red onion (60 g or 2.1 oz.)
- ✓ ½ cup chopped spring onion (40 g or 1.4 oz.)
- ✓ 1 cup sliced mushrooms (100 g or 3.5 oz.)
- ✓ ½ cup fresh basil leaves (10 g or 0.4 oz.)
- ✓ Salt and pepper, to taste
- ✓ Olive oil, for drizzling

Recipe:
1. Combine lukewarm water, honey or maple syrup, and yeast in a small bowl.
2. Let it sit for 5-10 minutes until it becomes frothy. In a large mixing bowl, combine flour and salt.

3. Make a well in the center and pour in the yeast mixture and olive oil. Stir until a dough forms.
4. Transfer the dough to a floured surface and knead for 5-7 minutes, until it is smooth and elastic. Place the dough in a lightly oiled bowl, cover it with a damp cloth or plastic wrap, and let it rise in a warm place for 1 to 1.5 hours, or until it doubles in size.
5. Preheat the oven to 475°F (245°C) and place a pizza stone or an upside-down baking sheet on the rack to heat.
6. In a pan, heat the olive oil, add the onion, and let it turn golden.
7. Then add the chopped mushrooms, spring onion, and basil. Then add the tomato sauce, crumbled tofu, crushed cashews, and nutritional yeast.
8. Allow the topping mixture to cook for 5 minutes, then set it aside to cool.
9. Once the dough has doubled in size, punch it down and transfer it to a floured surface. Roll the dough into your desired pizza shape and thickness.
10. Place the rounded dough on the heated baking sheet and bake for 15 minutes. Then, remove it from the oven and pour the topping over the slightly cooked pizza dough.
11. Allow the pizza to cook for 5-10 minutes until the crust is crispy.
12. Once baked, remove the pizza from the oven. Drizzle olive oil over the topping and sprinkle chopped fresh basil leaves on top.

13. Slice the pizza and serve it hot.

Total Nutritional Values of The Homemade Pizza with Tofu Cheese Recipe

Calories: 1400 Kcal
Protein: 35g
Carbohydrates: 200 g
Fat: 36 g
Fiber: 17g

Embrace The Young You

Homemade Nut Bar

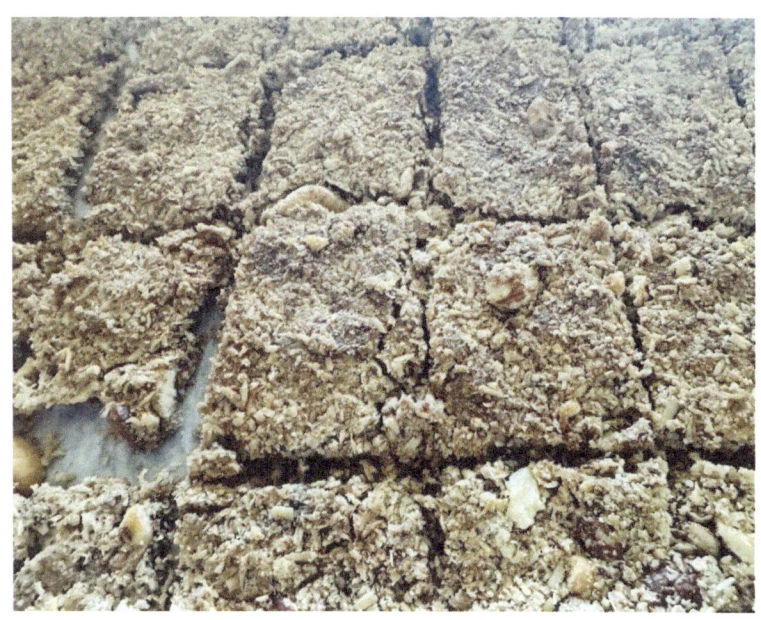

Preparation Time: 15-20 minutes
Cooking Time: 20-25 minutes
Serves: 12-16 bars

Ingredients:
- ✓ 1 cup organic rolled oats (90 g or 3.2 oz.)
- ✓ ½ cup shredded coconut (40 g or 1.4 oz.)
- ✓ ½ cup hazelnuts, chopped (60 g or 2.1 oz.)
- ✓ ½ cup cashew nuts, chopped (70 g or 2.5 oz.)
- ✓ ½ cup almonds, chopped (60 g or 2.1 oz.)
- ✓ ¼ cup almond flour (28 g or 1 oz.)
- ✓ ½ cup honey (170 g or 6 oz.) *or deseeded dates for a vegan option*
- ✓ ½ cup dates, chopped (75 g or 2.6 oz.)
- ✓ ¼ cup almond milk (60 ml or 2 oz.)
- ✓ 1 teaspoon vanilla extract (5 g or 0.1 oz.)
- ✓ ½ teaspoon ground cardamom (2.5 g or 0.08 oz.)

Recipe:
1. Preheat your oven to 350°F (175°C). Line a baking dish or tray with parchment paper.
2. Toast the oats and nuts by spreading the rolled oats, shredded coconut, hazelnuts, cashews, and almonds evenly in the prepared baking dish.
3. Toast in the oven for 8-10 minutes, or until lightly golden and fragrant. Keep an eye on them to prevent burning.
4. Remove from the oven and let them cool slightly.
5. Combine the toasted oats and nuts with almond flour in a large bowl.
6. Heat almond milk, vanilla extract, and ground

cardamom in a small saucepan over medium heat, stirring until well combined and heated through.
7. Take the milk off the heat and add a sweetener, such as honey or maple syrup, for a vegan option.
8. Pour the mixture over the oats and nuts.
9. Add the chopped dates and mix everything until evenly coated.
10. Transfer the mixture to the lined baking dish.
11. Press the mixture firmly and evenly into the oven dish using a spoon or spatula.
12. Bake in the preheated oven for 15-20 minutes, or until the edges turn golden brown.
13. Remove from the oven and let it cool completely.
14. Once cooled, cut the mixture into bars or squares with a sharp knife. Store them in an airtight container in the fridge or freezer for freshness.

Total Nutritional Values of The Homemade Nut Bar Recipe

Calories: 3300 Kcal
Protein: 80 g
Carbohydrates: 350 g
Fat: 210 g
Fiber: 45 g

Chocolate Delight Bites

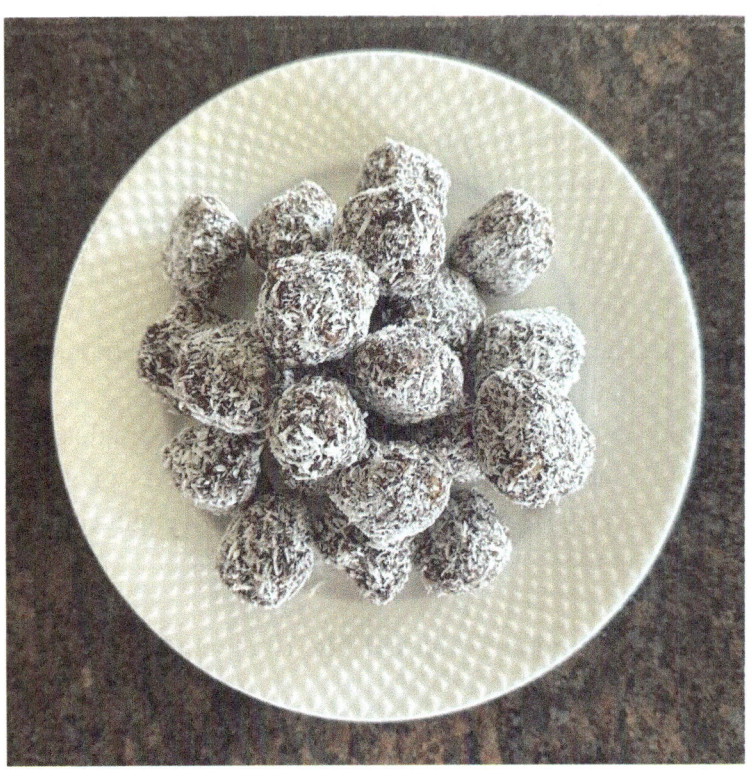

Preparation Time: 15 Minutes
Chilling Time: 30 Minutes
Total Time: 45 Minutes
Serves: 12 Truffles

Ingredients:
- ✓ 1 cup mixed nuts (almonds, cashews, and walnuts, finely chopped), 150 g or 5 oz.
- ✓ ¼ cup organic cocoa powder, 25 g or 1 oz.
- ✓ 1 teaspoon ground cinnamon, 5 g or 0.1 oz.
- ✓ 1 teaspoon vanilla extract, 5 g or 0.1 oz.
- ✓ ¼ cup coconut milk, 60 ml or 2 oz.
- ✓ ¼ cup coconut powder (optional for coating), 25 g (0.9 oz).
- ✓ 1 cup pitted dates (soaked in warm water for 10 minutes, then drained) 175 g or 6 oz.

Recipe:
1. In a food processor, pulse the mixed nuts until finely ground. Then transfer to a mixing bowl.
2. Combine the soaked dates, organic cocoa powder, ground cinnamon, vanilla extract, and coconut milk in the same food processor. Process until smooth, scraping down the sides of the bowl as needed.
3. Add the chocolate date mixture to the chopped nuts in the mixing bowl. Mix until well combined to form a sticky dough.
4. Using clean hands, roll small portions of the dough into bite-sized balls.
5. Roll the balls in coconut powder to coat them evenly.
6. Place the chocolate delight bites on a tray lined with parchment paper.
7. Chill in the refrigerator for at least 30 minutes to allow the mixture to firm.

8. Once chilled, transfer the chocolate delight bites to an airtight container and freeze them for freshness.

The recipe yields 20 bites.

Total Nutritional Values for The Chocolate Delight Bites Recipe

Calories: 1750 Kcal Protein: 45g Carbohydrates: 165g Fat: 115g Fiber: 40g

Embrace The Young You

Homemade Hummus

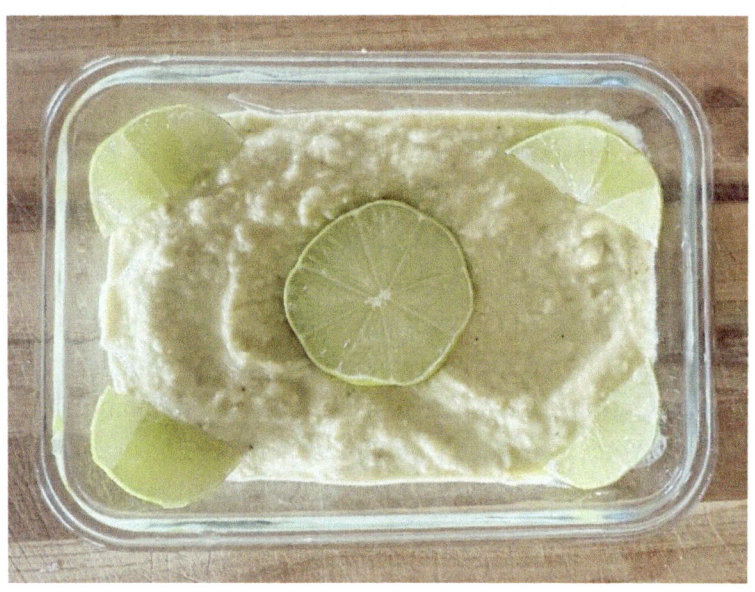

Preparation Time: 15 minutes
Cooking Time: No cooking time, using canned organic chickpeas
Serves: 6

Ingredients:
- ✓ 1 can of organic chickpeas (drained and rinsed) 450 g or 15 oz.
- ✓ ¼ cup tahini 25 g or 1 oz.
- ✓ ¼ cup fresh lemon juice (from 1 lemon)
- ✓ 3-4 small garlic cloves, minced
- ✓ 2 tablespoons extra-virgin olive oil 30 g or 1 oz.
- ✓ ¼ teaspoon turmeric 2 g
- ✓ ¼ teaspoon paprika 1.5 g
- ✓ Salt and pepper to taste
- ✓ 1 whole chili pepper (optional)
- ✓ Additional fresh lemon juice (2-3 as desired)
- ✓ Optional fresh herbs (such as parsley or cilantro)
- ✓ Water as needed (2-4 tablespoons for consistency)

Recipe:
1. In a food processor, combine chickpeas, tahini, lemon juice, minced garlic, olive oil, spices, chili, and salt and pepper.
2. Blend until smooth. If the hummus is too thick or chunky, add water a little at a time (1 tablespoon) until you reach the desired consistency.
3. Taste and adjust seasoning as needed.
4. Consider adding more salt or lemon juice, depending on your preference.
5. Adding herbs to hummus is optional.
6. Herbs like parsley and cilantro add extra flavor when used.

Total Nutritional Values of The Hummus Recipe

Calories: 819 Kcal Protein: 21 g Carbohydrates: 51 g Fat: 59 g Fiber: 12 g

Chickpeas are high in protein and fiber. Tahini, made from sesame seeds, is a good source of healthy fats and minerals. This dish is rich in folate, iron, magnesium, phosphorus, copper, and manganese. Garlic contains allicin, a sulfur-containing compound with numerous health benefits. Lemon juice is a good source of vitamin C. This dish can be used as a salad dressing, dip, or sandwich spread, and in soups, sauces, and stews to add flavor and fiber.

Total Nutritional Values for The Samosa Recipe Page (202)

Calories: 2900 Kcal Protein: 75 g Carbohydrates: 420 g Fat: 110 g Fiber: 55 g

Vegetarian Samosa

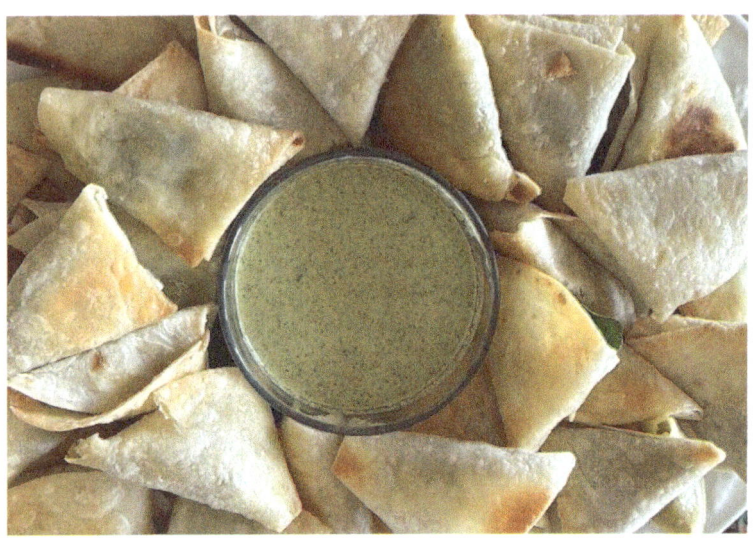

Preparation Time: 45 minutes
Cooking Time: 30 minutes
Serves: 20-30 Medium-sized samosa

Ingredients:

- ✓ 4-5 organic potatoes (medium size) 680 g or 20 oz.
- ✓ A packet of organic peas (frozen) 285 g or 10 oz.
- ✓ 2 medium-sized carrots, grated 140 g or 5 oz.
- ✓ 1 onion, diced 180 g or 6 oz.
- ✓ 1 teaspoon turmeric 5 g
- ✓ 1 teaspoon paprika 5 g
- ✓ 1 teaspoon curry powder 5 g
- ✓ 1 teaspoon dried cilantro (coriander) 5 g
- ✓ 1 cup chopped fresh coriander/cilantro 30 g or 1 oz.
- ✓ 1-2 lemon juice
- ✓ 1 teaspoon cayenne pepper 5 g
- ✓ 4-5 tablespoons olive oil 75 g or 2.5 oz.
- ✓ Salt and pepper to taste
- ✓ 1 serrano pepper (optional, if you like it hot)
- ✓ 5-6 cloves of garlic 60 g or 2 oz.
- ✓ 1 bag of organic tortillas (8-12 tortillas) - weighing 340-454 g or 12-16 oz.

Recipe:

1. Boil the potatoes in a medium-sized pot.
2. In a separate pan, bring the peas to a boil. Let the potatoes and peas cool.
3. Meanwhile, chop the onions. In a medium frying pan, heat the olive oil and fry the vegetables until golden brown.
4. Then, add the spices and the herbs. Let it cook for a few minutes, until you can smell the spices.

5. Next, peel the boiled potatoes and mash them in a large bowl. Then add the cooked peas and the remaining ingredients to the mashed potatoes.
6. Mix all the ingredients well. If you like it hot, add a serrano pepper.
7. Add the juice of one or two lemons and mix until well combined. Cut a tortilla in half. Place a spoonful of the potato and vegetable herb mixture on one half of the bread. Form a triangular cone by tucking in the side of the tortilla.
8. Repeat the process until all the mixture is used. Place the triangle samosas on an oven tray, drizzle with olive oil, and bake for 20-25 minutes at 350 °F, or until golden on both sides.
9. Enjoy cold or hot.

Homemade Accompaniment Sauce for Samosa
- ✓ 1 cup organic Greek yogurt (240 g or 8 oz).
- ✓ 2 cups chopped cilantro 60 g or 2 oz.
- ✓ 1 serrano pepper
- ✓ Juice of 1 whole lemon
- ✓ 2-3 cloves of garlic
- ✓ 1 teaspoon paprika
- ✓ Salt and pepper to taste

Mix all the ingredients in a food processor or mixer. Add water and lemon juice until you reach the desired consistency (neither too thick nor too runny). Serve with a platter of samosas. For the vegan option, use homemade hummus as the sauce.

Summary

Being young is a great life stage; generally, one tends to appreciate that phase of life after a few decades have passed. The sooner you adopt a holistic approach to well-being, the better that phase of your life will be. A holistic approach to well-being considers all aspects of our lives and health. It acknowledges that physical health, mental and emotional well-being, social connections, spiritual fulfillment, and environmental influences all play interconnected roles in our overall health and quality of life. By acknowledging all those aspects of our lives, we can feel and embrace youth in different decades. As mentioned earlier, physical health encompasses a healthy diet, regular physical activity, adequate sleep, and proper body care. It emphasizes preventive care and lifestyle choices that support long-term physical well-being. Mental and emotional well-being involves reducing stress, maintaining emotional resilience, and fostering positive mental health. Several practical techniques, such as mindfulness, music therapy, and stress-reduction practices, are incorporated into this aspect of the guidebook.

Social connections, relationships, and community support are crucial to well-being. Strong social connections can provide emotional support, reduce loneliness, and foster a sense of belonging. Spiritual fulfillment is closely tied to finding meaning and purpose in life. For some, it may include religious practices, while others find it in connection to the universe and nature, art, or personal growth.

Environmental factors, including air, water, and soil quality, can profoundly affect health and well-being. Lifestyle choices that can help improve well-being include avoiding harmful substances, practicing self-care, and engaging in activities that bring joy and fulfillment. It is interesting to note that younger generations, who are increasingly health-conscious and interested in non-alcoholic drinks, are driving demand for these products, and more companies are producing them for the market.

Integrating all aspects of well-being (physical, emotional, and mental) is essential. For example, physical exercise benefits the body and improves mood and mental clarity. A holistic approach to well-being emphasizes the interconnectedness of various aspects of life. It promotes health and happiness by addressing the whole person rather than focusing on isolated symptoms or concerns.

In this guidebook, I aim to empower you as you become independent and begin a new chapter of your life. Each chapter offers practical insights and actionable steps to help you navigate life's complexities and become the best version of yourself. In Chapter One, I discuss how to associate each phase of life's journey with different seasons. In Chapter Two, I present research findings from the literature on the transition to living away from home, including risk factors, for your general information. I provide solutions in the following chapters, accompanied by actionable steps. In Chapter Three, I discuss living away from home and embracing independence as an exhilarating journey of personal growth and self-discovery. However, it can also be daunting as you navigate the complexities of adulthood while striving to thrive holistically and pursue your purpose. I explain practical strategies and insights to help you flourish in your newfound independence. Chapter Four discusses practices for self-care, stress management, and maintaining balance in all areas of your life, fostering a sense of fulfillment and vitality. Healthy habits, such as regular exercise, a nutritious diet, adequate sleep, and stress-reduction techniques, are crucial for maintaining balance and overall well-being. The book emphasizes that prioritizing self-care is a non-negotiable part of one's routine. Chapter Five offers practical recipes for vegetarian and plant-rich vegan options, along with their nutritional values, as a practical guide toward a wellness journey.

I share the wisdom I've gained from my own experience and from watching my young adult children go through the same phase: being away from home, immigrating to another country to attend university, and starting independent lives. I also share my research findings in this field to help you discover independent lifestyles.

You are embarking on a path of self-discovery, and the sooner you find a well-trodden path that has been tested and shown to deliver desirable outcomes, the easier it will be to navigate obstacles. Of course, everyone is unique, and I want to emphasize that each individual appreciates their uniqueness.

One of the most important lessons from my life is that knowing you are enough at any stage is fundamental to bringing happiness, joy, and prosperity to yourself and those around you. The philosophers who emphasized the importance of knowing oneself realized centuries ago that we come into this world to discover ourselves. Reflect on the significance of living with purpose and meaning. Identify your passions and interests, align them with your values, and set meaningful goals that inspire you to make a positive impact on the world around you.

Our primary mission is to learn about ourselves and discover how unique we are. We learn lessons through life experience, or, as I call it, the school of life. I emphasize this message because I want you to realize your uniqueness at a young age, invest in yourself, and flourish by getting to know yourself so you can start a happy, prosperous life.

A significant amount of uncertainty exists around the world at any given time. One thing you can be sure of every day is that you can work on yourself to become a better version of yourself, one day at a time, without comparing yourself to anyone but yourself. Because we are all on this path through the wonderland of life, like Alice in Wonderland, you will make your own discoveries at your own pace. This life path can be beautiful from the outset, and the sooner you discover who you are and what you want from this brilliant life, the easier it becomes.

Self-reflection is a powerful practice for unlocking your true potential and living a more fulfilling life. You embark on self-discovery and personal growth by reflecting on your thoughts, feelings, and experiences. Whether through journaling, meditation, or introspective conversations, make self-reflection a regular part of your routine. Embrace the process with curiosity and compassion, knowing that the most significant insights often come from within.

Take the time to understand your strengths, weaknesses, values, and passions. Reflect on your goals and aspirations, and be honest about what truly matters to you. Self-awareness is the foundation of a fulfilling, purpose-driven life. As you get to know yourself and deepen your understanding of effective communication, you attract friends and build relationships with people who share your thoughts and perspectives. You also develop nurturing, healthy connections that enrich your life and support your growth.

I include a variety of plant-rich recipes that are easy to prepare, economical, and nutrient-dense. I have also included the nutritional information for the dishes for your reference. The primary reason for incorporating plant-based and vegetarian recipes into your diet is to introduce a variety of fruits, vegetables, pulses, nuts, and seeds. I also understand that some individuals are vegetarian or vegan for ethical reasons, and I respect that. When we realize our connection to nature, we become more mindful of what we put into it and what we take out of it.

So, my dear young people, at whatever age you are and wherever you live in the world, don't let the sad news around the globe distract you from your path of self-discovery. Your journey is uniquely yours, and the possibilities for growth and fulfillment are endless. I sincerely wish you a healthy and happy life, filled with all the blessings.

References

Abdel Magid, H., Milliren, C., Rice, K., Molanphy, N., Kennedy, R., Gooding, H., Richmond, T., Odden, M., & Nagata, J. (2022). Adolescent individual, school, and neighborhood influences on young adult hypertension risk. PLoS One, 17(4), e0266729.

2003. All you should eat: Fighting Freshman 15. *Food Service Director,* 16, 8:00-8:00.

Alkhalifah EAR, Alobaid AA, Almajed MA, Alomair MK, Al Abdul Adheem LS, Al-Subaie SF, Akbar A, Attimarad MV, Younis NS, Mohamed ME. Cardamom Extract Alleviates the Oxidative Stress, Inflammation, and Apoptosis Induced during Acetaminophen-Induced Hepatic Toxicity via Modulating Nrf2/HO-1/NQO-1 Pathway. Curr Issues Mol Biol. 2022 Nov 2;44(11):5390-5404. Doi: 10.3390/cimb44110365. PMID: 36354677; PMCID: PMC9688982.

2006. Changes in Body Weight and Fat Mass of Men and Women in the First Year of College: A Study of the Freshman 15. *Journal of American College Health,* 55, 41-46.

Aggarwal BB, Prasad S, Reuter S, Kannappan R, Yadav VR, Park B, Kim JH, Gupta SC, Phromnoi K, Sundaram C, Prasad S, Chaturvedi MM, Sung B. Identification of novel anti-inflammatory agents from Ayurvedic medicine for prevention of chronic diseases: "reverse pharmacology" and "bedside to bench" approach. Curr Drug Targets. 2011 Oct;12(11):1595-653. Doi: 10.2174/138945011798109464. PMID: 21561421; PMCID: PMC3170500.

Al-Huwailah, A., Abdelsattar, M., Al-Hamdan, N., Derar, E., Alazmi, S., & Griffiths, M. (2023). Empathic Skills Training as a Means of Reducing Cyberbullying among Adolescents: An Empirical Evaluation. International Journal of Environmental Research and Public Health, 20(3), 1846.

Alshammari, G., Alsulami, T., & Al-Nouri, D. (2022). Phenolic Compounds, Antioxidant Activity, Ascorbic Acid, and Sugars in Honey from Ingenious Hail Province of Saudi Arabia. Applied Sciences, 12(16), 8334.

Ambra R, Lucchetti S, Pastore G. A Review of the Effects of Olive Oil Cooking on Phenolic Compounds. Molecules. 2022 Jan 20;27(3):661. Doi: 10.3390/molecules27030661. PMID: 35163926; PMCID: PMC8838846.

Anderson, D. A., Shapiro, J. R., & Lundgren, J. D. 2003. The first year of college is a critical period for weight gain: An initial evaluation. *Eating Behaviors,* 4, 363-367.

Auti ST, Kulkarni YA. Neuroprotective Effect of Cardamom Oil Against Aluminum-Induced Neurotoxicity in Rats. Front Neurol. 2019 Apr 30;

10:399. Doi: 10.3389/ fneur. 2019.00399. PMID: 31114535; PMCID: PMC6502995.

Babajide A, Ortin A, Wei C, Mufson L, Duarte CS. Transition Cliffs for Young Adults with Anxiety and Depression: Is Integrated Mental Health Care a Solution? J Behav Health Serv Res. 2020 Apr;47(2):275-292. Doi: 10.1007/s11414-019-09670-8. PMID: 31428923; PMCID: PMC7028507.

Bailey, T. A. (2015). The Effects of Social Norms Feedback on Fruit and Vegetable Consumption and Skin Carotenoids Among College Students. https://doi.org/10.26076/73ed-0cfb

Bartel L, Mosabbir A. Possible Mechanisms for the Effects of Sound Vibration on Human Health. Healthcare (Basel). 2021 May 18;9(5):597. doi: 10.3390/healthcare9050597. PMID: 34069792; PMCID: PMC8157227.

Basso M, Zorzan I, Johnstone N, Barberis M, Cohen Kadosh K. Diet quality and anxiety: a critical overview of the gut microbiome. Front Nutr. 2024 May 15; 11:1346483. doi: 10.3389/fnut.2024.1346483. PMID: 38812941; PMCID: PMC11133642.

Becker, C., Schumacher, C., Beck, K., Tschan, F., Semmer, N., Hochstrasser, S., Marsch, S., & Hunziker, S. (2020). Association of self-esteem, personality, stress, and gender with resuscitation team performance: A simulation-based study. PLoS One, 15(5), e0233155.

Benefits of olive oil Archives - Green Press.
https://greenpress.ca/tag/benefitsofoliveoil/
Benefits of Holistic Medicine for Addiction Treatment.
https://www.amethystrecovery.org/4-benefits-of-holistic-medicine-for-addiction-treatment/.
Bleidorn W, Arslan RC, Denissen JJ, Rentfrow PJ, Gebauer JE, Potter J, Gosling SD. Age and gender differences in self-esteem: a cross-cultural window. J Pers Soc Psychol. 2016 Sep;111(3):396-410. doi: 10.1037 /pspp0000078. Epub 2015 Dec 21. PMID: 26692356.
Borzì AM, Biondi A, Basile F, Luca S, Vicari ESD, Vacante M. Olive Oil Effects on Colorectal Cancer. Nutrients. 2018 Dec 23;11(1):32. doi: 10.3390/nu11010032. PMID: 30583613; PMCID: PMC6357067.
Botanical Extracts: Natural Recovery for Strenuous Exercise. https://silentbio.com/botanical-extracts-recovery-strenuous-exercise/.
Brady LS, Herkenham M. Candace B Pert. Neuropsychopharmacology. 2013 Dec;38(13):2730. doi: 10.1038/npp 2013.269. Epub 2013 Nov 12. PMCID: PMC3828549.
Bright Partner Spotlight | OrangeWip. https://cola.orangewip.com/editions/october-2023-mental-health-awareness/partner-spotlight-bright-marketing

Brown, C. 2008a. The "Freshman 15" information trail systematically reviews a health myth within the research and popular literature. *Health Information & Libraries Journal*, 25, 1-12.

Calabrese, F., Calabrese, F., Calabrese, F., Celano, G., Celano, G., Riezzo, G., Ignazzi, A., Sila, A., De Nucci, S., Rinaldi, R., Linsalata, M., Vacca, M., Apa, C., De Angelis, M., Giannelli, G., De Pergola, G., Russo, F., & Russo, F. (2023). Metabolomic Profiling of Obese Patients with Altered Intestinal Permeability Undergoing a Very Low-Calorie Ketogenic Diet. Nutrients, 15(24), 5026.

Candace B. Pert, Molecules of Emotion: The Science Behind Mind-Body Medicine (Touchstone, New York) 1999.

Castelló A, Boldo E, Amiano P, Castaño-Vinyals G, Aragonés N, Gómez-Acebo I, Peiró R, Jiménez-Moleón JJ, Alguacil J, Tardón A, Cecchini L, Lope V, Dierssen-Sotos T, Mengual L, Kogevinas M, Pollán M, Pérez-Gómez B; MCC-Spain Researchers. Mediterranean Dietary Pattern is Associated with Low Risk of Aggressive Prostate Cancer: MCC-Spain Study. J Urol. 2018 Feb;199(2):430-437. doi: 10.1016/j.juro.2017.08.087. Epub 2017 Aug 23. PMID: 28842246.

Centers for Disease Control, C. 2010. Healthy Campus 2010 *In* Survey (1988-1994), N. C. F. H. S. N. H. A. N. E. (ed.). www.acha.org [accessed July 2011].

Chin, K.Y., & Ima-Nirwana, S. (2016). Olives and Bone: A green Osteoporosis Prevention Option. International Journal of Environmental Research and Public Health, 13(8), 1-11.

Cianciosi D, Forbes-Hernández TY, Afrin S, Gasparrini M, Reboredo-Rodriguez P, Manna PP, Zhang J, Bravo Lamas L, Martínez Flórez S, Agudo Toyos P, Quiles JL, Giampieri F, Battino M. Phenolic Compounds in Honey and Their Associated Health Benefits: A Review. Molecules. 2018 Sep 11;23(9):2322. doi: 10.3390/molecules23092322. PMID: 30208664; PMCID: PMC6225430.

Choi Y, Choi SH, Yun JY, Lim JA, Kwon Y, Lee HY, Jang JH. The relationship between levels of self-esteem and the development of depression in young adults with mild depressive symptoms. Medicine (Baltimore). 2019 Oct;98(42): e17518. doi: 10.1097/MD.0000000000017518. PMID: 31626112; PMCID: PMC6824750.

Chomsky, N. (2006). *Language and Mind*, Cambridge University Press.

Chopra, D. 2004. *The Book of Secrets: Unlocking the hidden dimensions of your life, Random House Large Print.*

Christopher Moore, Socrates and Self-Knowledge (Cambridge: Cambridge University Press, 2015).

Community Interventions: A Brief Overview and Their Application to the Obesity Epidemic | Journal of Law, Medicine & Ethics | Cambridge Core.

https://www.cambridge.org/core/journals/journal-of-law-medicine-and-ethics/article/abs/community-interventions-a-brief-overview-and-their-application-to-the-obesity-epidemic/448335E8B6(Pyridoxine)EE073819AFED6CDE0DD0EC.

Comini S, Mandras N, Iannantuoni MR, Menotti F, Musumeci AG, Piersigilli G, Allizond V, Banche G, Cuffini AM. Positive and Negative Ions Potently Inhibit the Viability of Airborne Gram-Positive and Gram-Negative Bacteria. Microbiol Spectr. 2021 Dec 22;9(3): e0065121. doi: 10.1128/Spectrum 00651-21. Epub 2021 Nov 10. PMID: 34756075; PMCID: PMC8579920.

Crombie Aaron, P., Ilich Jasminka, Z., Dutton Gareth, R., Panton Lynn, B., & Abood Doris, A. 2009. The freshman weight gain phenomenon revisited. *Nutrition Reviews,* 67, 83-94.

Cultivating Resilience: Building Inner Strength to Overcome Life's Challenges. https://www.mindandbodyfitness.org/post/cultivating-resilience-building-inner-strength-to-overcome-life-s-challenges.

Czenczek-Lewandowska, E., Czenczek-Lewandowska, E., Leszczak, J., Wyszyńska, J., Baran, J., Weres, A., & Lewandowski, B. (2022). The Role of Physical Activity in the Reduction of Generalized Anxiety Disorder in Young Adults in the Context of the COVID-19 Pandemic. International Journal of

Environmental Research and Public Health, 19(17), 11086.

David, M. C., Edward, L. G., & Jesse, M. S. 2003. Why Have Americans Become More Obese? *Journal of Economic Perspectives,* 17, 93-118.

Determinants of fruit & vegetable and fat intake in university students: a cross-sectional explanatory study | Scriptiebank. https://www.scriptiebank.be/scriptie/2013/determinants-fruit-vegetable-and-fat-intake-university-students-cross-sectional.

Drugs and Lactation Database (LactMed®) [Internet]. Bethesda (MD): National Institute of Child Health and Human Development; 2006-. Brewer's Yeast. [Updated 2023 Sep 15].Available from: https://www.ncbi.nlm.nih.gov/books/NBK572248/.

Dunne, C. & Somerset, M. 2004. Health Promotion in Universities: What Do Students Want? *Health Education,* 104, 360-370.

Escrich E, Solanas M, Moral R, Costa I, Grau L. Are olive oil and other dietary lipids related to cancer? Experimental evidence. Clin Transl Oncol. 2006 Dec;8(12):868-83. doi: 10.1007/s12094-006-0150-5. PMID: 17169760.

Esmond, S., Healy, D., Cabral, G., & Larsen, J. (2012). The Challenges at Chartwells. https://core.ac.uk/download/47189684.pdf

Finding Joy in Your Job: Embracing Fun Along Your Career Path – Rhizome Consulting. https://rhizomeng.com/2023/08/23/can-work-be-fun-unlocking-the-joy-in-your-professional-journey.

Fraleigh, S. (2000). Consciousness Matters. https://core.ac.uk/download/233569039.pdf/.

Freud, S. (1924). *A general introduction to psychoanalysis*, trans. Joan Riviere.

Eating for your bones: The most essential nutrients for your bone health in menopause and beyond. - My Menopause Transformation. https://www.mymenopausetransformation.com/bone-health/eating-for-your-bones-the-most-essential-nutrients-for-your-bone-health-in-menopause-and-beyond/

Galisteo M, Duarte J, Zarzuela A. Effects of dietary fibers on disturbances clustered in the metabolic syndrome. *J Nutr Biochem*. 2008; 19:71–84. [PubMed] [Google Scholar].

Gebauer JE, Göritz AS, Hofmann W, Sedikides C (2012) Self-Love or Other-Love? Explicit Other-Preference but Implicit Self-Preference. PLoS ONE 7(7): e41789. https://doi.org/10.1371/journal.pone.0041789

Gebauer JE, Göritz AS, Hofmann W, Sedikides C (2012) Self-Love or Other-Love? Explicit Other-Preference but Implicit Self-Preference. PLoS ONE 7(7): e41789. https://doi.org/10.1371/journal.pone.0041789.

https://www.healthymepa.com/2018/05/15/4-benefits-self-love-important/. 4 benefits of self-love and why it is essential, revised December 14th, 2022, accessed January 2024.

Gittelsohn, J. & Kumar Mohan, B. 2007. Preventing childhood obesity and diabetes: Is it time to move beyond the school? *Pediatric Diabetes,* 8, 55-69.

Gooding HC, McGinty S, Richmond TK, Gillman MW, Field AE. Hypertension awareness and control among young adults in the National Longitudinal Study of Adolescent Health. Journal of General Internal Medicine. 2014;29(8):1098–1104. [PMC free article] [PubMed].

Gordon-Larsen P, Adair LS, Nelson MC, Popkin BM. Five-year obesity incidence in the transition period between adolescence and adulthood: The National Longitudinal Study of Adolescent Health. American Journal of Clinical Nutrition. 2004;80(3):569–575. [PubMed]

Gortmaker, S. L., Swinburn, B. A., Levy, D., Carter, R., Mabry, P. L., Finegood, D. T., Huang, T., Marsh, T. & Moodie, M. L. 2011. Changing the future of obesity: science, policy, and action. *The Lancet,* 378, 838-847.

Gutiérrez-González, E., Castelló, A., Fernández-Navarro, P., Castaño-Vinyals, G., Llorca, J., Salas-Trejo, D., Salcedo-Bellido, I., Aragonés, N., Fernández-Tardón, G., Alguacil, J., Gracia-Lavedan, E., García-Esquinas, E., Gómez-Acebo, I., Amiano, P.,

Romaguera, D., Kogevinas, M., Pollán, M., & Pérez-Gómez, B. (2019). Dietary Zinc and Risk of Prostate Cancer in Spain: MCC-Spain Study. Nutrients, 11(1), 18.

Ha, Eun-Jeong et al., Effect of Nutrition Intervention Using a General Nutrition Course for Promoting Fruit and Vegetable Consumption among College Students - Journal of Nutrition Education and Behavior. https://www.jneb.org/article/S1499-4046(08)00755-0/fulltext.

Howland RH. Vagus Nerve Stimulation. Curr Behav Neurosci Rep. 2014 Jun;1(2):64-73. doi: 10.1007/s40473-014-0010-5. PMID: 24834378; PMCID: PMC4017164.

Hubert, H. B., Eaker, E. D., Garrison, R. J., & Castelli, W. P. 1987. Lifestyle Correlates of Risk Factor Change in Young Adults: An Eight-Year Study of Coronary Heart Disease Risk Factors in The Framingham Offspring. *American journal of epidemiology*, 125, 812-831.

Imamura F, Micha R, Khatibzadeh S, Fahimi S, Shi P, Powles J, Mozaffarian D; Global Burden of Diseases Nutrition and Chronic Diseases Expert Group (NutriCoDE). Dietary quality among men and women in 187 countries in 1990 and 2010: a systematic assessment. Lancet Glob Health. 2015 Mar;3(3): e132-42. doi: 10.1016/S2214-109X (14)70381-X. PMID: 25701991; PMCID: PMC4342410.

Irazusta, A., Hoyos, I., Irazusta, J., Ruiz, F., Diaz, E. & GIL, J. 2007. Increased cardiovascular risk associated with poor nutritional habits in first-year university students. *Nutrition Research,* 27, 387-394. Jacka FN. Nutritional psychiatry: where to next? *EBioMedicine.* 2017 Mar; 17:24–29. doi: 10.1016/j.ebiom.2017.02.020. https://linkinghub.elsevier.com/retrieve/pii/S2352-3964(17)30079-8. [PMC free article] [PubMed] [CrossRef] [Google Scholar].

Jacka FN. Nutritional psychiatry: where to next? *EBioMedicine.* 2017 Mar; 17:24–29. doi: 10.1016/j.ebiom.2017.02.020. https://linkinghub.elsevier.com/retrieve/pii/S2352-3964(17)30079-8. [PMC free article] [PubMed] [CrossRef] [Google Scholar].

Jackal, R. K. (2010). Psychological and Behavioral Correlates of Freshman BMI Change. https://core.ac.uk/download/70419703.pdf.

Jiang SY, Ma A, Ramachandran S. Negative Air Ions and Their Effects on Human Health and Air Quality Improvement. Int. J. Mol. Sci. 2018 Sep 28;19(10):2966. doi: 10.3390/ijms19102966. PMID: 30274196; PMCID: PMC6213340.

Jiménez-Sánchez, A., Jiménez-Sánchez, A., Piñar-Gutiérrez, A., & Pereira-Cunill, J. (2022). Therapeutic Properties and Use of Extra Virgin

Olive Oil in Clinical Nutrition: A Narrative Review and Literature Update. Nutrients, 14(7), 1440.

Jukanti AK, Gaur PM, Gowda CL, Chibbar RN. The nutritional quality and health benefits of chickpea (Cicer arietinum L.): a review. Br J Nutr. 2012 Aug;108 Suppl 1: S11-26. Doi: 10.1017/S0007114512000797. PMID: 22916806.

(2015). Investing in The Health and Well-Being of Young Adults.

Kawachi I, Berkman LF. Social ties and mental health. J Urban Health. 2001 Sep;78(3):458-67. doi: 10.1093/jurban/78.3.458. PMID: 11564849; PMCID: PMC3455910.

Kessler RC, Chiu WT, Demler O, Walters EE. Prevalence, severity, and comorbidity of 12-month DSM-IV disorders in the National Comorbidity Survey Replication. Archives of General Psychiatry. 2005;62(6):617–627. [PMC free article] [PubMed].

Konstantinidi M, Koutelidakis AE. Functional Foods and Bioactive Compounds: A Review of Its Possible Role in Weight Management and Obesity's Metabolic Consequences. Medicines (Basel). 2019 Sep 9;6(3):94. doi: 10.3390/medicines6030094. PMID: 31505825; PMCID: PMC6789755.

Larson, N., Neumark-Sztainer, D., Laska, M. N., & Story, M. 2011. Young Adults and Eating Away from Home: Associations with Dietary Intake Patterns and Weight Status Differ by Choice of Restaurant. *Journal of the American Dietetic Association,* 111, 1696-1703.

Laska, M. N., Pasch, K. E., Lust, K., Story, M., & Ehlinger, E. 2009. Latent Class Analysis of Lifestyle Characteristics and Health Risk Behaviors among College Youth. *Prevention Science,* 10, 376-386.

Lawag IL, Lim LY, Joshi R, Hammer KA, Locher C. A Comprehensive Survey of Phenolic Constituents Reported in Monofloral Honeys around the Globe. Foods. 2022 Apr 15;11(8):1152. doi: 10.3390/foods11081152. PMID: 35454742; PMCID: PMC9025093.

Lee, P.Y., Ong, T.A., Muna, S., Alwi, S. A. R. S. & Kamarudin, K. 2010. Do university students have high cardiovascular risk? A pilot study from. *Malaysian Family Physician,* 5, 41-43.

Lee, S., & Lee, E. (2020). Effects of Cognitive Behavioral Group Program for Mental Health Promotion of University Students. International Journal of Environmental Research and Public Health, 17(10), 3500.

Levitsky, David A. & Youn, T. 2004. The More Food Young Adults Are Served, the More They Overeat. *Journal of Nutrition,* 134, 2546-2549.

Lloyd-Richardson, E. E., Bailey, S., Fava, J. L., & Wing, R. 2009a. A prospective study of weight gain during the first and second college years. *Preventive Medicine,* 48, 256-261.

Major BC, Le Nguyen KD, Lundberg KB, Fredrickson BL. Well-Being Correlates of Perceived Positivity Resonance: Evidence from Trait and Episode-Level Assessments. Pers Soc Psychol Bull. 2018 Dec;44(12):1631-1647. doi: 10.1177/0146167218771324. Epub 2018 May 13. PMID: 29756547; PMCID: PMC8750237.

Mandal D, Sarkar T, Chakraborty R. Critical Review on Nutritional, Bioactive, and Medicinal Potential of Spices and Herbs and Their Application in Food Fortification and Nanotechnology. Appl Biochem Biotechnol. 2023 Feb;195(2):1319-1513. doi: 10.1007/s12010-022-04132-y. Epub 2022 Oct 11. PMID: 36219334; PMCID: PMC9551254.

Markellos, C., Gavriatopoulou, M., Halvatsiotis, P., Sergentanis, T., & Psaltopoulou, T. (2022). Olive oil intake and cancer risk: A systematic review and meta-analysis. PLoS One, 17(1), e0261649.

Matud MP, Díaz A, Bethencourt JM, Ibáñez I. Stress and Psychological Distress in Emerging Adulthood: A Gender Analysis. J Clin Med. 2020 Sep 4;9(9):2859. Doi: 10.3390/jcm9092859. PMID: 32899622; PMCID: PMC7564698.

McMacken M, Shah S. A plant-based diet for the prevention and treatment of type 2 diabetes. J

Geriatr Cardiol. 2017 May;14(5):342-354. doi: 10.11909/j.issn.1671-5411.2017.05.009. PMID: 28630614; PMCID: PMC5466941.

Mediterranean Dietary Pattern is Associated with Low Risk of Aggressive Prostate Cancer: MCC-Spain Study - ibs. Granada. https://www.ibsgranada.es/articulos/mediterranean-dietary-pattern-is-associated-with-low-risk-of-aggressive-prostate-cancer-mcc-spain-study/

Mihalopoulos, N. L., Auinger, P., & KLEIN, J. D. 2008. The Freshman 15: Is it Real? *Journal of American College Health,* 56, 531-534.

Mine Y. Egg proteins and peptides in human health--chemistry, bioactivity and production. Curr Pharm Des. 2007;13(9):875-84. doi: 10.2174/138161207780414278. PMID: 17430187.

Minkler, M. 2000. Using Participatory Action Research to Build Healthy Communities. *Public Health Rep.,* Mar-Jun; 115, 191–197.

Moral R, Escrich E. Influence of Olive Oil and Its Components on Breast Cancer: Molecular Mechanisms. Molecules. 2022 Jan 12;27(2):477. Doi: 10.3390/molecules27020477. PMID: 35056792; PMCID: PMC8780060.

Morshed MB, Saha K, De Choudhury M, Abowd GD, Plötz T. Measuring Self-Esteem with Passive Sensing. Int Conf Pervasive Comput Technol Healthc. 2020 May; 2020:363-366. doi:

10.1145/3421937.3421952. Epub 2020 May 18. PMID: 34350057; PMCID: PMC8329846.

More energy – Abundance Academy. https://myabundanceacademy.ca/tag/more-energy/.

Moser MB, Rowland DC, Moser EI. Place cells, grid cells, and memory. Cold Spring Harb Perspect Biol. 2015 Feb 2;7(2): a021808. Doi: 10.1101/cshperspect. a021808. PMID: 25646382; PMCID: PMC4315928.

Nakayama H, Tsuge N, Sawada H, Masamura N, Yamada S, Satomi S, Higashi Y. A single consumption of curry improved postprandial endothelial function in healthy male subjects: a randomized, controlled crossover trial. Nutr J. 2014 Jun 28;13:67. Doi: 10.1186/1475-2891-13-67. PMID: 24972677; PMCID: PMC4082484.

Nelson, M. C., Kocos, R., Lytle, L. A., & Perry, C. L. 2009. Understanding the Perceived Determinants of Weight-related Behaviors in Late Adolescence: A Qualitative Analysis among College Youth. *Journal of Nutrition Education and Behavior,* 41, 287-292.

Nie, Y. Y., Zhou, L. J., Li, Y. M., Yang, W. C., Liu, Y. Y., Yang, Z. Y., Ma, X. X., Zhang, Y. P., Hong, P. Z., & Zhang, Y. (2022). Hizikia fusiforme functional oil (HFFO) prevents neuroinflammation and memory deficits evoked by lipopolysaccharide/aluminum trichloride in zebrafish. Frontiers in Aging Neuroscience, (), n/a.

Nguyen QC, Tabor JW, Entzel PP, Lau Y, Suchindran C, Hussey JM, Halpern CT, Harris KM, Whitsel EA. Discordance in national estimates of hypertension among young adults. Epidemiology. 2011;22(4):532–541. [PMC free article] [PubMed].

Nguyen QC, Whitsel EA, Tabor JW, Cuthbertson CC, Wener MH, Potter AJ, Halpern CT, Killeya-Jones LA, Hussey JM, Suchindran C, Harris KM. Annals of Epidemiology. 2014. [October 22, 2014]. (Blood spot-based measures of glucose homeostasis and Diabetes prevalence in a nationally representative population of young U.S. adults). (published online ahead of print). http://dx.doi.org/10.1016/j.annepidem.2014.09.010. [PMC free article] [PubMed].

O'Day, Danton. (2017). First Artists of the Rubaiyat of Omar Khayyam, Vol. I-III.

Olas, B. (2022). Bee Products as Interesting Natural Agents for the Prevention and Treatment of Common Cardiovascular Diseases. Nutrients, 14(11), 2267.

Okouchi, R., Shuang, E., Yamamoto, K., Ota, T., Seki, K., Imai, M., Ota, R., Asayama, Y., Nakashima, A., Suzuki, K., & Tsuduki, T. (2019). Simultaneous Intake of Euglena Gracilis and Vegetables Exerts Synergistic Anti-Obesity and Anti-Inflammatory

Effects by Modulating the Gut Microbiota in Diet-Induced Obese Mice. Nutrients, 11(1), 204.

Olas, B. (2022). Bee Products as Interesting Natural Agents for the Prevention and Treatment of Common Cardiovascular Diseases. Nutrients, 14 (11), 2267.

OpenAI. (2023). *ChatGPT* (September 25 Version) [Large language model]. https://chat.openai.com.

Oso, A. A., & Ashafa, A. O. (2021). Nutritional Composition of Grain and Seed Proteins. https://doi.org/10.5772/intechopen.97878.

Osumanu, H., Choy, Y., & Jalloh, M. (2021). Chemical and Biological Characteristics of Organic Amendments Produced from Selected Agro-Wastes with Potential for Sustaining Soil Health: A Laboratory Assessment. Sustainability, 13(9), 4919.

Orth U., Robins R.W., Roberts B.W. Low self-esteem prospectively predicts depression in adolescence and young adulthood. *J. Pers. Soc. Psychol.* 2008; 95:695–708. doi: 10.1037/0022-3514.95.3.695.

Paffenbarger, R. S. & Wing, A. L. 1969. Chronic Disease in Former College Students. *American journal of epidemiology,* 90, 527-535.

Palenzuela-Luis N, Duarte-Clíments G, Gómez-Salgado J, Rodríguez-Gómez J.A., Sánchez-Gómez MB. International Comparison of Self-Concept, Self-Perception, and Lifestyle in Adolescents: A Systematic Review. Int J Public Health. 2022 Sep

29; 67:1604954. doi: 10.3389/ijph.2022.1604954. PMID: 36250150; PMCID: PMC9556634.

Palmberg, A. (2015). Use and Perspectives of a Social Marketing Campaign to Improve Fruit and Vegetable Intake. https://doi.org/10.25772/RZT0-TA17.

Papathanasopoulos A, Camilleri M. Dietary fiber supplements: effects in obesity and metabolic syndrome and relationship to gastrointestinal functions. Gastroenterology. 2010 Jan;138(1):65-72. e1-2. doi: 10.1053/j.gastro.2009.11.045. Epub 2009 Nov 18. PMID: 19931537; PMCID: PMC2903728.

Pauwels EK, Volterrani D, Mariani G, Kostkiewicz M. Mozart, music and medicine. Med Princ Pract. 2014;23(5):403-12. doi: 10.1159/000364873. Epub 2014 Jul 19. PMID: 25060169; PMCID: PMC5586918.

Pearlin L.I., Lieberman M.A., Menaghan E.G., Mullan J.T. The stress process. *J. Health Soc. Behav.* 1981; 22:337–356. doi: 10.2307/2136676.

Pyne, L. (2015). Eat well, run better! Women's Fitness, (139) 65-66.

Pereira, M. A., Kartashov, A. I., Ebbeling, C. B., VAN HORN, L., SLATTERY, M. L., JACOBS, D. R. & LUDWIG, D. S. 2005. Fast-food habits, weight gain, and insulin resistance (the CARDIA study): a 15-year prospective analysis. *Lancet (British edition),* 365, 36-42.

Petrella C, Di Certo MG, Gabanella F, Barbato C, Ceci FM, Greco A, Ralli M, Polimeni A, Angeloni A, Severini C, Vitali M, Ferraguti G, Ceccanti M, Lucarelli M, Severi C, Fiore M. Mediterranean Diet, Brain and Muscle: Olive Polyphenols and Resveratrol Protection in Neurodegenerative and Neuromuscular Disorders. Curr Med Chem. 2021;28(37):7595-7613. doi: 10.2174/0929867328666210504113445. PMID: 33949928.

Pop LM, Iorga M, Iurcov R. Body-Esteem, Self-Esteem and Loneliness among Social Media Young Users. Int J Environ Res Public Health. 2022 Apr 21;19(9):5064. doi: 10.3390/ijerph19095064. PMID: 35564458; PMCID: PMC9104843.

PSYCH-K - Bruce H. Lipton, https://www.brucelipton.com/psych-k-2/.

Racette, S. B., Deusinger, S. S., Strube, M. J., Highstein, G. R., & Deusinger, R. H. 2005. Weight Changes, Exercise, and Dietary Patterns During Freshman and Sophomore Years of College. *Journal of American College Health,* 53, 245-251.

Racette, S. B., Deusinger, S. S., Strube, M. J., Highstein, G. R., & Deusinger, R. H. 2008. Changes in Weight and Health Behaviors from Freshman through

Senior Year of College. *Journal of Nutrition Education and Behavior,* 40, 39-42. Reflecting on Our Journey: Wrapping Up 2023 with 5 Tips for a Positive Transition - I Am Valerie Hatcher. https://valeriehatcher.com/aging-with-grace-style-podcast/reflecting-on-our-journey-wrapping-up-2023-with-5-tips-for-a-positive-transition/.

Rizzo G, Baroni L. Soy, Soy Foods and Their Role in Vegetarian Diets. Nutrients. 2018 Jan 5;10(1):43. doi: 10.3390/nu10010043. PMID: 29304010; PMCID: PMC5793271.

Robert. M. Williams, WPSYCH-K... The Missing Piece/Peace in Your Life. (Myrddin Publications), January 1, 2013.

Rodríguez-Sánchez, L., López-Abente, G., Núñez, O., & Pollán, M. (2019). Different spatial patterns of municipal prostate cancer mortality in younger men in Spain. PLoS One, 14(1), e0210980.

Roncero-Martín R, Aliaga Vera I, Moreno-Corral LJ, Moran JM, Lavado-Garcia JM, Pedrera-Zamorano JD, Pedrera-Canal M. Olive Oil Consumption and Bone Microarchitecture in Spanish Women. Nutrients. 2018 Jul 26;10(8):968. doi: 10.3390/nu10080968. PMID: 30049982; PMCID: PMC6115724.

Seitz NN, Lochbühler K, Atzendorf J, Rauschert C, Pfeiffer-Gerschel T, Kraus L. Trends in Substance Use and Related Disorders: Analysis of the Epidemiological Survey of Substance Abuse, 1995-

2018. Dtsch. Arztebl Int. 2019 Sep 2;116(35-36):585-591. doi: 10.3238/arztebl.2019.0585. PMID: 31587706; PMCID: PMC6804271.

Salehi, B., Azzini, E., Zucca, P., Varoni, E., Anil Kumar, N., Dini, L., Panzarini, E., Rajkovic, J., Peluso, I., Mishra, A., Nigam, M., Setzer, W., Polito, L., Iriti, M., Sureda, A., Quetglas-Llabrés, M., Martorell, M., Martins, N., Sharifi-Rad, M., . . . Sharifi-Rad, J. (2020). Plant-Derived Bioactives and Oxidative Stress-Related Disorders: A Key Trend towards Healthy Aging and Longevity Promotion. Applied Sciences, 10(3), 947.

Sekoni, O., Mall, S., & Christofides, N. (2022). The relationship between protective factors and common mental disorders among female urban slum dwellers in Ibadan, Nigeria. PLoS One, 17(2), e0263703.

Sin NL, Rush J, Buxton OM, Almeida DM. Emotional Vulnerability to Short Sleep Predicts an Increase in Chronic Health Conditions Over 8 Years. Ann Behav Med. 2021 Nov 18;55(12):1231-1240. doi: 10.1093/abm/kaab018. PMID: 33821929; PMCID: PMC8824788.

Shamsuddeen, S. B., Epuru, S., Syeda, B. F., & Al Rashedi, W. F. M. (2014). Risk Factors for Obesity among Saudi Female College Students. https://core.ac.uk/download/249333761.pdf

Shetty, V., Hamza, M., Ahmed, A., Shirlal, S., & Kumar, M. (2020). Coping Behaviors in Economically

Disadvantaged Hostel Students in India. Indian Journal of Health and Wellbeing, 11(4-6), 213-215.

Sreedharan S, Nair V, Cisneros-Zevallos L. Protective Role of Phenolic Compounds from Whole Cardamom (*Elettaria cardamomum* (L.) Maton) against LPS-Induced Inflammation in Colon and Macrophage Cells. Nutrients. 2023 Jun 29;15(13):2965. doi: 10.3390/nu15132965. PMID: 37447289; PMCID: PMC10346154.Stoll, D. (2023).

Strong, K. A., Parks, S. L., Anderson, E., Winett, R., & Davy, B. M. (2008). Weight Gain Prevention: Identifying Theory-Based Targets for Health Behavior Change in Young Adults. *Journal of the American Dietetic Association,* 108, 1708-1715.e3.

Soto-Madrid D, Pérez N, Gutiérrez-Cutiño M, Matiacevich S, Zúñiga RN. Structural and Physicochemical Characterization of Extracted Proteins Fractions from Chickpea (*Cicer arietinum* L.) as a Potential Food Ingredient to Replace Ovalbumen in Foams and Emulsions. Polymers (Basel). 2022 Dec 27;15(1):110. doi: 10.3390/polym15010110. PMID: 36616460; PMCID: PMC9824673.

Swinburn, B. A., Sacks, G., Hall, K. D., McPherson, K., Finegood, D. T., Moodie, M. L., & Gortmaker, S. L. 2011. The global obesity pandemic: shaped by global drivers and local environments. *The Lancet,* 378, 804-814.

Szcześniak, M., Szcześniak, M., Falewicz, A., Strochalska, K., & Rybarski, R. (2022). Anxiety and Depression in a Non-Clinical Sample of Young Polish Adults: Presence of Meaning in Life as a Mediator. International Journal of Environmental Research and Public Health, 19(10), 6065.

Taboada, P., Taboada, P., Coelho, A., & Coelho, A. (2023). The Southern European Atlantic Diet and Its Supplements: The Chemical Bases of Its Anticancer Properties. Nutrients, 15 (19), 4274.

The Annie E. Casey Foundation, 2023 Population Estimates, U.S. Census Bureau. The young adult population is ages 18 to 24, according to race and ethnicity.

Tuck KL, Hayball PJ. Major phenolic compounds in olive oil: metabolism and health effects. J Nutr Biochem. 2002 Nov;13(11):636-644. doi: 10.1016/s0955-2863(02)00229-2. PMID: 12550060.

Vella-Zarb, Rachel, A. & Elgar, Frank, J. 2010. Predicting the "Freshman 15": Environmental and Psychological Predictors of Weight Gain in First-Year University Students. *Health Education Journal,* 69, 321-332.

Vilaro, M., Colby, S., Riggsbee, K., Zhou, W., Byrd-Bredbenner, C., Olfert, M., Barnett, T., Horacek, T., Sowers, M., & Mathews, A. (2018). Food Choice Priorities Change Over Time and Predict Dietary Intake at the End of the First Year of College Among Students in the U.S. Nutrients, 10(9), n/a.

Wang, S., Reed, D. B., Goli, S., & Goswami, D. 2011. Blood leptin and C-reactive protein provide a more sensitive assessment than blood lipids and other inflammatory biomarkers in overweight university students. *Nutrition Research,* 31, 586-593.

Weber I, Sienko A, Urban A, Szwed C, Czajkowski K, Basta P, Sienko J. Relationship between the gut microbiome and endometriosis and its role in pathogenesis, diagnosis, and treatment: a systematic review. Ginekol Pol. 2023 Oct 2. doi: 10.5603/gpl. 97581. Epub ahead of print. PMID: 37772919.

Wengreen HJ, Moncur C. Change in diet, physical activity, and body weight among young adults during the transition from high school to college. Nutr J. 2009 Jul 22; 8:32. doi: 10.1186/1475-2891-8-32. PMID: 19624820; PMCID: PMC2720988.

Whatnall MC, Hutchesson MJ, Sharkey T, Haslam RL, Bezzina A, Collins CE, Tzelepis F, Ashton LM. Recruiting and retaining young adults: what can we learn from behavioral interventions targeting nutrition, physical activity, and obesity? A systematic review of the literature. Public Health Nutr. 2021 Dec;24(17):5686-5703. doi: 10.1017/S1368980021001129. Epub 2021 Mar 16. PMID: 33722332; PMCID: PMC10195641.

Wohns, R. N. W. (2020). Editorial. What doesn't kill you makes you stronger. Neurosurgical Focus FOC, 49(5), E4. https://doi.org/10.3171/2020.8.FOCUS20763.

Zheng J, Zheng S, Feng Q, Zhang Q, Xiao X. Dietary capsaicin and its anti-obesity potency: from mechanism to clinical implications. Biosci Rep. 2017 May 11;37(3): BSR20170286. Doi: 10.1042/BSR20170286. PMID: 28424369; PMCID: PMC5426284.

Zhu C, Sawrey-Kubicek L, Beals E, Rhodes CH, Houts HE, Sacchi R, Zivkovic AM. Human gut microbiome composition and tryptophan metabolites were changed differently by fast food and Mediterranean diet in 4 days: a pilot study. Nutr Res. 2020 May; 77:62-72. Doi: 10.1016/j.nutres.2020.03.005. Epub 2020 Mar 26. PMID: 32330749.

Made in the USA
Las Vegas, NV
17 February 2026